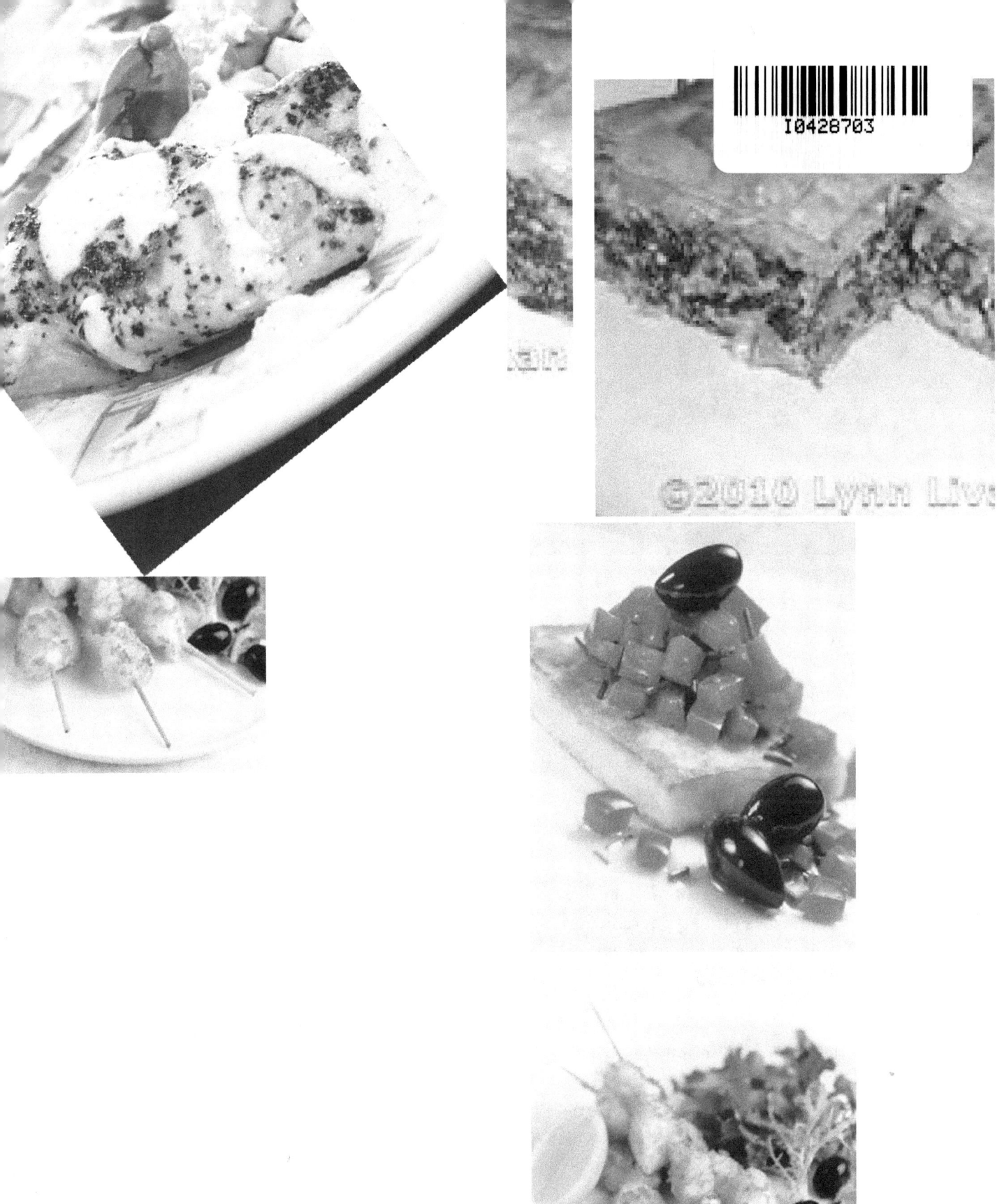

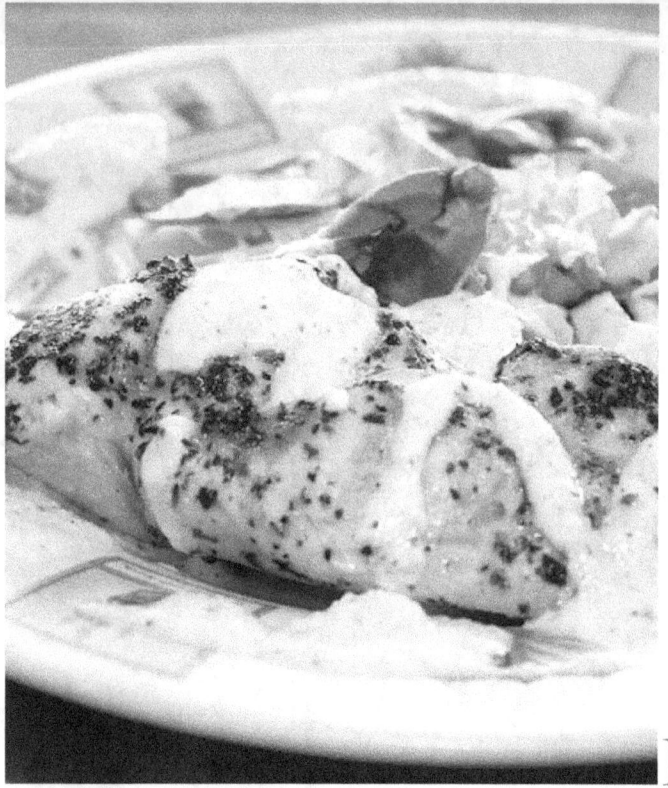

Mediterranean diet and lifestyle.

Introduction

The Mediterranean diet is about lifestyle first and diet second.

This name is just a misappropriation of the correct meaning.

Mediterranean diet projects images and fantasies of the Mediterranean scenery, but most importantly conveys images of nature, of balance and of seasonal regular produce that accentuates the added appreciation of the culinary experience of all the herbs, the vegetables of all the produce that the region provides.

To become healthier you need to become the philosopher, rediscovering your connection to nature, learning and appreciating vegetables and fruits and how they can be added in cooking to accentuate taste and how you can apply them in your daily eating routine so that you ensure your daily nutritional requirements which are imperative to lose weight, are met.

I remember reading a book about a monk teaching his student about the miracle of life and all its offspring and how every flower and herb has a name.

What a difference a pizza makes when you add basil to that tomato and boccachini?

Therein lies the heart of appreciating food and the culinary experience therein.

Unfortunately when you see paradise and how all of nature sustained us physically and spiritually and then witness the stark contrast and the frightening reality of agribusiness prevalent today and in our corporatised food chain then, you start to really appreciate this by gone era, when food was not a commodity but was sacred , it comprised an integral part of our cultural traditional existence that sustained cultures and communities to live in balance and harmony and it was a time where even the desserts contained natural ingredients that kept your waistline. Food was produced in season, was fresh and therefore preserved its nutrients. People often got together and helped prepare dishes so to ensure that people ingested a variety of foods, especially the salads and vegetables prepared as a delicious cooking recipe dish. people would be truly replenished and satisfied without having to spend the energy on their own to meticulously and obsessionally find the right kind and proportion of food that suits their difficult and unmaintainable artificial diet regime.

These fad diets focus on deficiency and repression without taking into account the guidance of preparing a diet regime that is feasible, practical and nutritionally beneficial. These criteria of preparing food dishes is imperative because if the body is not replenished properly nutritionally, then you cannot be healthy and if you cannot be healthy, you would not be able to lose weight and sustain weight loss in perpetuity.

Before the addition of fat causing chemicals and hormones were manufactured in canned and processed foods, nature sustained all and guided how, when and what we should eat according to the natural metabolistic clock that ticks inside us and according to season availability. They represented to primary ingredients of our diet. Like potatoes and rice are staple diets, the cucumber and tomato crops ensured the salad variety. When consumed in combination, satisfaction of your appetite ensured and harmony of diet and lifestyle intake was achieved. The gathering and collecting of these crops ensured an exercise that formed an important and crucial element to village culture as it entailed exercise and togetherness of family in their efforts to procure the right ingredients harvested for the right nutritious dish at the dinner table.

By nature and intuitively we respond to this indispensable quest and thirst for knowledge regarding our total well being. It is infused in our very make up and consciousness and just like how everyone, without fail, loves to walk in parks and loves the scenery that relaxes them and especially those that love preparing their own food in gardening, so to everyone should love how an apple keeps the doctor away, how an apple is a powerful antioxidant that maintains our immune system so that we keep healthy and functional. How garlics and onions clean food and provide additional benefit as they accentuate taste in our food.

How the use of garlics, onions, chilis, ginger root burn fat and also clean our bodies so we are healthier and more energetic and even better how they even compliment the taste in your salads. Don't we want to be in control of our own healths or do we want to rely submissively to doctors prescriptions which at times can do more harm than good because of their frequent collusion with pharmaceutical companies that represent conflicts of interests. Maybe your someone that passively submits to a doctors prognosis without any question. Everyone has a freewill. Don't your know your weight is related to your health?

Health is a holistic reality and the Mediterranean experience essentializes this reality.

That nothing changes. Principles in nature remain the same and our needs remain the same and as the world becomes more polluted, all the more we need to be more wary and conscious of the foods we ingest. To bring up issues of health and medicine is imperative to holistically address diet issues. It is area the dieting market segment would not impinge as authors of this industry have more than satisfied their legal obligation by merely regurgitating diet tactic and fade taboos and recipes and successfully avoided the more important dimensions to weight loss. By not at least taking it into account, it can distort the solution and goal of what we trying to set out and achieve.

It is not just that unnecessary medication is detriment to your weight but this is inseparably connected to your general health. Hence this is the angle of this book addressing the root cause of weight gain with the telescope and visor of lifestyle and perspective. Perspective is viewing life in a philosophical manner, eg. The ability to discern eating places, to understand food politics and how food take out are primarily concerned with overhead and so are more likely to resort to cheaper grade oil. This provides the intellectual and emotional incentive motive to attempt at least to eat more at home or at least be wary when eating out. Lazy people do not take the extra effort in finding a good eat place. A good gauge of course is if after you have eaten the food you feel a bloat or some stress or illness that occurs as a result of eating at the premise. Always a keep a note.

The solution to our weight issues lies in a new reorientated perspective of your lifestyle views and choices. Drinking coffee at right time in the day, drinking instead of eating, avoiding the cake with the coffee and have a piece of bread instead. Eating just a piece of fruit in the morning before you go off in the day etc etc.

In evaluating the nature of things, the bodies propensity to enjoy desserts is marginal to what unhealthy people actually take. It is not natural. They do so because it becomes a passion of which they have lost control and find confidence in sponging up all their sorrows through the lone pursuit of excessive food consumption.

We cannot change our basic integral needs, but we can place it into its proper functioning state of operation. When one is consumed for example with reading or working, then the tendency to resort to dessert to fulfil an urge is reduced as their occupation, activity in lifestyle effectively replaces this urge and alleviates any pressure that may drive them for relief through the intake of food. This is food intake mechanics and it is universal and true everywhere.

So food is replaced with a soul food that is life and satisfaction is therefore found. Unhealthy overweight people rarely deep down enjoy eating junk food as it has become a habit and the binging habit therefore lost its novelty of anticipation where the self justified and natural urge that abstinence from it creates and of which amplifies the enjoyment of the dessert or junk food is lost.

By nature if you were to have junk all day,you will still be hungry because you did not consume the proper foods in adequate proportions. This is why eating after desserts after dinner is beneficial, especially when we learn to adapt by adding fruit to icecream-- compliments the food while at the same time is more healthier. This little step makes a difference to little steps throughout the day and therein you find a realised lifestyle that works without the pressure and exertion of forcing yourself into unrealistic crash diets.

The only time you may force yourself is fasting, which is valuable for your body and when your sick, you are forced to reflect on what your eating and make the correct readjustment of your food intake for the sake of your health. That is why the stomach growing bigger huge after unfortunate eating experience and leads to us worrying of our looks can be used as a positive and a defence mechanism which justifiably keeps us in check and just alone on its own premise by moderating and taming this force will see a positive health building lifestyle emerge to form its basic rugged edges until you refine it with other little activities and exercises which are spontaneous and without exertion or maximising the output per energy you put in. which equals a believable and practicable and realisable diet loss schedule incorporating true to life tested steps to achieve it.

Contemporary society has altered this picture perfect state, although never perfect, we live in an age of excess, of over indulgence, of an age where we get our food from 2 major food corporations that do not provide natural produce freshly delivered, but store them in cans with added preservatives and market them and control and marginalise the farmers that do produce natural product without the additives of chemicals.

But you can still reach homeostasis or a balanced state of health by actively sorting and filtering information and actively engaged in health building activities that only means better moods, better feelings of happiness. We all want to reach a state of euphoria when we go out with friends and so red wine does the trick, but did not the broccoli you had during the day also provide the extra impetus for you to reach this ecstatic state? Well this information provides you with the motivation to eat broccoli raw, how easier it is when it is combined in a recipe preparation?

2 process of elimination

Lets get right to it we all love to binge. It within itself relaxes us and it is ok to feel weak and resort to it. But we also need to be aware of how our emotional states induce us into this activity and one has to be prepared for the consequences and therein lies the motivation to refrain from binging for at least another week because of the guilt of that occasion when we did. These mechanics within itself provide a natural equilibrium that resemble a balanced rhythmic graph replicating close to the balanced lifestyle you need to achieve.

eg. it is natural to refrain from a certain food and try to rid the feeling by making a little note and promise to yourself to at least avoid the food for another month.

So it you did it 12 times in the year, your average gain of your health is still positive and therefore balance is achieved despite these anomalies. But maybe these anomalies provide the valuable experience in your life that sustains a positive lifestyle because these occasions of bad binging provides the motivation to do it better the next time around or at least it may provides an impetus to slowly improve year by year by incorporating in your lifestyle additional health promoting activities which have relatively little exertion and disruption to your day while keeping and even building your energy in the day and therefore maximise your satisfaction.

You can then moderate this with drinking water instead of softdrink. Enjoy the experience of slow cooked sunflower chips whilst enjoying the occasion as relatively minor obstruction to your lifestyle goal objectives.

A Suggestion vege chips in sunflower oil, 40% less fat than regular chips.

Without even starting , getting rid of certain foods in diet does allot without building pressure of always watching what you eat.

The process of elimination is a powerful start to your new discovery and your new lifestyle objectives. It can be half the work

This can be a new awakening, learning articles about the role of trans fatty acids and which oils have them. Is powerful avoidance behaviour integrated into your new lifestyle.

Building the right alternatives to them is essential to building new behaviours and habits that are health promoting.

Some guides as follows-

Eat More seafood less meat.

More vegetarian dishes. There are many that are just as enjoyable as meat ones.

No more processed cheese, more feta haloumi style cheeses

Always check in the burgers to take the fat off the bacons

Compensation behaviours after a bad eating experience. A quick detox{ a major lifestyle imperative}, more on this latter

Develop the right habits and you can still binge.

When you binge—buy small packet of chips, preferably with sunflower oil and always drink purified water to wash it down and you will enjoy this occasional binge more.

If you have a beautiful pasta dish for lunch, have a lighter dinner meal to compliment this regime as this comprises the sensible approach to diet and lifestyle for your long term health.

If you suppress your body by not eating, firstly this does not make you lose weight, as you need energy , so eat well but eat diversely.

 Though veging out should be minimised and mitigated, in a balanced day of moderate but fulfilling eating, these episodes of binging have no effect on their own right in accumulating weight, as your new found balanced dieting and lifestyle will naturally cancel and iron out any discrepancies to the norm and therefore your metabolism views it as merely an anomaly and therefore you still go on to score weight loss point in the day an with relatively little exertion. This is the maintainable, realistic and practical approach to weight loss is contentment with your lifestyle and outlook without wasting your time watching the weight clock go down, only having to build up pressure and completely give up on your diet loss exercise.

Giving your more confidence and an impetus to indulge in your favourite foods without feeling guilty that you will gain weight.

 But we are all human.

The fad diets totally miss this point, It is about long term averaging and consolidation and compensation within a lifestyle frame where you are oblivious to your efforts.

Also very important – speak a little latter-- the importance of harnessing your taste and appreciation of vegetable foods through a re education program, usually in the form on learning to cook culinary dishes which combine vegetables into a enjoyable and tasteful experience.

Avoid the following.

Packaged food is one of the major reasons for obesity in the 21st century.

Fast food and chips contain trans fatty acids. For example when buying chips, Find the alternative vege chip varieties as they contain better oils than the mainstream brands.

Avoid cooked chips when eating out as they use oils that are full of trans fatty acids. Especially avoid take away places. You may want to eat something to fill your appetite but with fast food places it is not even worth the occasional binge, as these foods more than likely would subject you to a food poisoning episode because of all the chemicals used in the process of making the foods. These foods disrupt your stomach enzymes which find it difficult to digest this food and this leads to an immediate elevation of cholesterol.

Now if we must take that burger and you are planning to compensate for it latter on, instead of chips have salad with it and wash it with water as then the anti oxidants in the salads will cancel out the fattening and metabolistic disrupting effects of the burger.

Many articles illuminate this one area, so substantial, that we eliminate it and discipline ourselves to avoid, we are talking a 30% head start.

Understanding the nature of oils, especially those marketed as canola. Unintentionally leads us into an area that inadvertently makes us as philosophers and label readers and researchers. The ability to Look behind the marketing labels and discerning the real nutritional benefit of foods that we buy and controlling our passions by habitualising the eating of good foods{and the ability to enjoy the} is an imperative requirement of our healthy lifestyle routine. Many eat an apple for example , not because of the taste, but because of a sense of accomplishment and a sense of doing good for their body and also because it replenishes and refreshes us and makes our mouth all clean. Eating food is not just taste, but a lifestyle meaning eating for health, eating for replenishment between breaks and eating so we are energized for the day. This requires perspective and culture, where no longer is food merely about taste and instant gratification but is also a health promoting force which performs a function more important that merely gratifying your taste buds. This is why presuming the clothes of a philosophy is indispensable to achieving desired weight loss.

If you need that fast food break, always have it without chips and try to drink 100 percent orange juice. However when in the middle of the night, there is nothing, inhabit discipline and be abstinent for the duration of night is highly rewarding. Nuts and dried fruits can be a little snack alternative mixed with ginger lollies. A great snack in the middle of the night, try tomatoes basil and boccachini in extras virgin olive oil and crispy bread. If you eat excessively in the night, then always conduct a little detox by eating some fruit. This is the law of accomodation and self reflection. Also it is the law of frugality. Eating excessively leads to living life in excess that leads to unhappiness and a sense of continuous dissatisfaction.

However if you make that late night trip to the petrol station, make it an infrequent occurrence and make each time a guilt experience to prevent you from doing it again for at least a month. Never ever induce yourself to throw up--- this will not make you learn, but you have habitualised a highly dangerous and unbeneficial act that does not address the root issue of our excess consumption. The bloative feelings we get at times, are mostly chemicals, the best thing to do is the clean your system out with filtered water with some basil and honey infused or some peppermint tea. If still a bit upset, do a little exercises, but remember you are looking for the long term average. So bear with it-- it is a learning experience and remember we are only human and we make mistakes. Because sooner or latter we are going to have something that does not agree with us-- this just builds resistance and character in us and helps to concentrate our efforts along better lines.

This is the learning experience curve where we incrementally improve ourselves through trial and error and bad experiences, so do not be afraid to be weak and have faith.

Still within this frame you can achieve balance. Perhaps eliminating the habit all together. But never store junk food in cupboards.

25% orange juices and soft drinks do not replenish your thirst anyway,they make you more bloaty. Make sure orange juices are 100 percent and are freshly squeezed. The difference to your energy and health levels,as a result, are immeasurably beneficial. A simple act with exponential benefits is the way you ought to view things.

Stay away from Cheddar cheese.

Just eliminating this food goes along way, understanding the process by which they make this industrial sludge, will show you how much your body's metabolism has to work the effects off. One small behavioural action with an immeasurable negative consequence.

Not just bloating, but the effects are often a sticky perspiring feeling and they also reduce the quality of your complexion. They affect your mood and how you feel and add a bulge with it.

This knowledge reaffirmed on its own, should act as a wake up motivational device where we reflect before engaging in a bad behavioural activity how the little value gained from satisfying a taste bug cannot be compared to the negative effects made as a result of its consumption.

 ok. If you need to have cheddar cheese have it in a platter with tomato and cucumber and maybe garlic. This act will accentuate the taste while the vegetables in a delicious combination will cancel out the negatives of the ingredients within the cheese.

Taking responsibility for our actions, helps us further engage and make better decisions for our health and weight, our feelings and complexion.

Better still red wine with crackers and blue cheese. The only cost is the extra money to buy better quality cheese.

Cheddar cheese left in the sun, will show you the transfatty oil coming out of it.

I heard that the product is close to black and the yellow is simply dye with plenty of salt on it. It is a food with virtually no nutritional value as the food is dead sludge.

If this is a regular feature of your diet then certainly by abstaining totally from this food would improve your health substantially and therefore improve your weight.

Better alternatives are fetta haloumi and boccacini cheese

The role of marketing in food—fad diets

I will only outline a brief note in this area, however it is a very important one to further study and consider.

Fast food diet schemes are all marketing fades trying to profit from the huge dieting industry. All try to promote the magical convenient and instantaneous solution to weight problem.

By virtue of being marketable accessibly,they have to also portray the ease and "without inconvenience approach of their magical dieting method so that it sells numbers and people find their total solution in the one product.

In consequence people are inadvertently moved away from the real cause of their eating issues and into ones that are totally unrealistic and difficult to maintain as they do not address underlining issues and causes of the problem.

One needs to discern between real information and the information wrapped up as a marketing package with disclaimers and claims. This is significant!

The role of the media in influencing behaviour and perceptions about meat for example.

The meat industry says that to have sufficient intakes of iron you must have meat 3-4 times a week. One in examining the truth to the matter we realise that meat can contribute to cancer because of all the hormones and chemicals added to the meat and that in fact there are many alternative vegetarian foods that provide use with protein –such as beans.

A recent harvard study has illuminated us how bad meat is to your health

Of course this is an educational informative lesson about the role of marketing to create perceptions that are unfounded, about the nutritional value of food.

The Mediterranean diet has the witness, testimony and experience of the nice elegant weightless girl, often portrayed in the media with beautiful complexion who diets predominately on fish, salad and vegetables. Not excessive consumptions of meat. Meat is not bad in moderation.

The Mediterranean diet is an example of a diet that encompasses a lifestyle.

Firstly the importance of family getting together and sharing food.

People getting together is healthy within itself. A common observed effect of this can be seen how drinking wine with company accentuates the properties of the wine to a more enjoyable effect. Also the nutrition of the food you eat and its health affects is both accentuated and complimented when you eat it while sitting in the sun and by the beach than sitting alone in a 4 wall room by yourself.

When your eating food outdoors in the mediterranean garden with family and friends, you are making the most the experience, your eyes are tantalised and inspired by the views and the harmony the garden evokes with your well being. Your picking basil in the garden so that you can enjoy your tomato and crispy bread and olives even more, which by the way, this is merely snacking. When you rather snack on these natural delights rather than many of the other artificial food, then you know you are on your way to a better diet so forgive your brother and sister and carefully choose your friends. A know its not a definite science.

 The air provides the vital phegma or vital oxygen important for your mood and digestion and your general well bring and the wine bring you closer to ecstasy per lower proportion of its consumption than if you were to have it indoors or by yourself.

The company and laughter makes you forget about your cold and your are spontaneously healed by the whole experience you have engaged in.

everyone knows how better we feel when we are around others and in good company.

This is the reason for the continual success of cinemas and the reason people love going to cafes. The reason why tele marketing centres are barely sustainable.

People power and people working in teams provide the atmosphere for optimising work efficiency in work places as there is unseen communal bond where the energies of people bounce off each other and so as a result energy is increased exponentially .

This same dynamic applies to eating with company in a scenic destination, this is the meaning to a healthy lifestyle. Not eating in sterile and clinically uninspiring places.

 Drinking red wine with food is a lifestyle trait not a diet or recipe.

With relative ease and comfort accompanied by your 5 course of mezes, the dessert and coffee all in the outdoor setting of family and friends with the nurturing summer breeze.

This is not something that should be out of your way, although initially changing habits might be hard, but by reconditioning through effort it is attainable.

The best diets are not the ones repackaged as miracle wonders that will improve you over night, they are the cultural traditional dishes, whereby by virtue of eating set recipe dishes, you are abstaining from all the other garbage, as well as all the other fades promoting short term solutions with short sighted ideologies.

Mainly because it is not a diet but a lifestyle outlook of appreciating the taste of vegetables and salads mixed in with fish and even meat occasionally.

Acquiring a taste for how vegetables compliment the taste of food, not only broadens your horizons culturally, whereby you become a more conscientious eater, but you will also became a little philosopher, understanding the medicinal properties of foods, so to better learn about your body and health and take charge of your health in an age of pharmaceutical sponsored medical centres. If you are a little sick. Add benefit to your salad by adding more ginger and onion and balsamic oil-- this bean salad will satisfy your appetitive with fat free bread. You are satisfied because you have been nutritionally replenished-- the two concepts are mutually exclusive and intrinsically linked. This is a major reason for excess eating, this is because processed food does not have the nutritional content and so therefore we continue to be hungry and eat unnecessarily. eg. When you eat cakes and sweets, does not quench your appetite until you have a cooked and warm meal filled with nutrients.

The problem of obesity, is not an issue of diet but also lifestyle outlook and being informed about foods by self criticising/{critiquing and monitoring} your eating food habits in an age of processed food, will change your attitude towards maintaining your holistic health and therefore weight as a viable long term solution.

It may be an effort in the beginning, however once you tailor the right habits to your new outlook on life, then you will be lighter for it and then you will enjoy your occasional short breads and ice cream pancake snacks because you are accustomed to your new diet lifestyle routine and confident that the averaging off effect will counter compensate for any occasional excess trans fat interplaying in your diet. But as rarely as we have these sweets—they are also important because it is good we reward ourselves and truly enjoy our sweets as a let loose and to unwind every so often—otherwise repressing ourselves through excessive control with out a natural organic rhythmic existence will make us completely rebel our routine. Which by the way is at ease because we by acquiring a taste for the better foods we are oblivious to those occasions when we miss eating the junk food.

But when you do have something that disagrees with you, by listening to your body, then make that experience an opportunity by motivating you next time to avoid that particular course or ingredient of food.

What all chefs know is how the garlics, onions, shallots and gingers all add to the taste of foods and incidentally your health.

If you love gardening, your love nature and if you love nature then you love natural foods and appreciate their role in your daily intake regime.

Now many people do not realise that all these foods are powerful anti toxin and anti cancerous foods that prevent illness and maintain your immune system and metabolism.

The reason why the medicinal and philosophical health aspects are primarily focused in this thesis, is to emphasis the point that losing weight is everything to do with your state and the condition of your health.

There are no short cuts, and by following extreme diets of abstaining from food for long periods of time or by excessively eating too many salads and soups, only aggravates your appetite and effects your clarity and direction in life. It is about proportional balance.

Remember it is ok to feel full, this is your body's message, you need energy to lose weight and when you are content and eating the right foods with occasional binges and mistakes, that is a good sign..

As we learn and even when we still do the same mistakes, we eventually, through persistence, build that resolution and conviction to not go to all those junk food chains for at least 3- 6 months and see how you feel then.

Sometimes it takes you to eat something so bad that it makes you feel guilty not because it is fattening, but because of how it makes us feel, we know it to be unhealthy, so we should be ever so vigilant at any of these opportune trigger points to reorientate a new outlook and all the more reason to employ immediate little detoxes after these events. This can be triggered by realising that your favourite junk food place makes you feel whisy and lethargic and slightly dizzy? Is it worth it? Lets channel our anger to positives and bring about a revitalised and refreshed view to these situations.

I am not talking about when you had a good steak and vegetables and had some nice wine and you feel full. This is very good. BUT NOW EAT FRUIT AND OR GELLATO –your digestion is your cleaner and restorer .

Your body needs the nutrition.

One of the tricks is, when your really hungry and the only shops that are open are the junk food places, just remember, try to go temper and moderate yourself and go through a bit of pain for a rewarding outcome and an important opportunity to avoid an act with regretful consequences.

Be patient and walk another block to that thai place, where at least the food is delicious and contains the nutritional value through the vegetables, even though the oils and salts at times contained in them are questionable. Or simply wait til you get home. Perhaps the learning experience here is to have ensured a nutritional meal by preparing something in advance so to avoid this future pit hole.

One of the main features of the Mediterranean lifestyle is the ability to cook and to enjoy cooking your own food. This obviously requires the habit of visiting fresh food markets everyday and waking up 30 minutes earlier before going to work.

Remember this valuable reflector y exercise replaces the gathering from harvest exercise in traditional days and so we need to reflect on food culture, think of economical ways to cook food that is both affordable and healthy and save plenty of money in the process and avoiding food places that cook with bad recycled oils. This means organising your kitchen and spending the priority and time to store and place food for easy retrieval when preparing and cooking food.

It is important to pace yourself with your routine and schedule, so as not to abandon yourself in front of a luring fast food chain because of hunger pains.

Taking lunch with you. By making the food is a great way to go so that you can control the good olive oil you put in ,as well as adding in a little bit of locally produced garlic as a preventive antedote to all the smog and pollution we may face during the day. { note garlic overseas are bleached, gassed and irradiated}. If you do not live in australia, always buy local regional garlic because they do not go through this chemical irradiating process

detox

People get caught up with the notion that a detox is something you set out to do once every so often and involves absolute hardship and deprivation, its thought of as requiring allot of effort to plan the day and completely disrupt your normal eating routine.

This is not entirely true. It is true that detox requires us to avoid our usual intake of foods for a certain amount of time but it is not something that is separate to our daily routine to the extent that it is foreign and when we finish our detox we plunge ourselves in again to our unhealthy diet lifestyle , especially over toxifying ourselves with alcohol beverages on the weekend without learning about how the blend of spirits and fresh fruits gives us the buzz but also ensures a relatively healthy and spirited evening without the heavy toxic effects of straight up cheap alcohol and beer and its not doing well on your complexion either..

Detox is continuous in the lifestyle diet. This means whenever we have fruit and a little bit of gellato after dinner, this is a little detox. When we had a softdrink and want to clean our bodies with filtered water---so to properly replenish our thirst,this is a small detox.

In the course of a week they add up to a more effective detox than one that entails a complete and sudden deprivation that are the hallmarks of diet fads eating patterns.

In the Mediterranean diet context this means after dinner we have plenty of fruit and share it.

It means salads with everything we eat act as little detox agents constantly renewing our system while satisfying properly our appetites.

When we add extra chilis or onions to our salad so to clean and compensate for a bad food choice earlier in the day, this is another detox. So detoxing does not necessarily always mean abstaining from certain foods over a prolonged amount of time and infrequently done. It is continuously done and perpetually beneficial to your diet and lifestyle and important to building our propensity and toleration to eating occasional questionable nutritionally limited foods like hamburgers for example.

As a result, your metabolism increases and your balance maintained.

This sends envy to your friends who wonder how you eat so much yet never put on weight. This is also because after the pizza you are going to have tea and how you plan to moderate you next meal in balanced proportion,not to mention you good eating behaviours already mentioned.

Eating a hamburger or pizza can be nutritional and this eating to hearts content in invaluable in your lifestyle diet routine because without replenishment and sustenance, there is no health and without health there is no slim figure.{ slim does not mean those unusually thin models on the catwalk}

An important example of frequent detox in the med diet lifestyle plan is having filtered water with your coffee-- compensating for the strength of a coffee with water.

Additionally Coffee should never have too much milk.

However because we have it in our mind of a once off binge free detox day, we tend to get lazy and neglect every other given day. Detox should be done in small packets and doses and done regularly and perpetually and you will notice when done in this way, there is little pain or effort as your detoxes are dispersed in series of small little packets throughout the course of your day. This little exertion and little disruption to your normal lifestyle pattern makes this a believable, achievable and practical lifestyle weight loss adaptation.

Like eating fruit after a meal is a form of detox,{as mentioned} already neutralising the overwhelming food content in your belly by aiding digestive process and the capacity for your body to extract more sustenance from your food content eaten and propensity to reject the impurities and unwanted by products in the food.

A small thing goes along way, as when we do small things everyday, they amount to the total picture state and story of a better outlook and more adaptable and flexible immune system.

This is more in consensus and synchronization to your body's natural rhythmic cycles which are governed by your immune and metabolism systems through your digestive system and all the organs carrying out their delegated tasks to achieve the body in a primo balance.

Listening to the direction of the body is imperative, especially when we eat something we became guilty of and something that subsequently we regret.

Reciprocal effect

When this occurs, we all say at some point," well I eat all this crap now, what is another burger or chips going to do" we say to ourselves?

The answer is that we get caught up in this reciprocal destructive effect with the expectant results being that there is never a time or place to eat well because we are waiting or silently and agonisingly preparing to make that sudden and extreme detox day to get rid of our guilt accumulated throughout the month. Instead of detoxing without effort and obliviously through a series of frequent and small detoxes throughout the day after a meal, we incrementally condition ourselves that, "since we ate something bad,I'll keep doing so until on sunday when I completely purge and go on a crash detox and fast.

Firstly the sudden and immediate detox you do after weeks of a big binge,being in case example the sunday, would have a sling shot effect. Since the body is not incrementally used to fasts /detox, this fast is a complete anomaly with very small or little influence on you lo\sing weight for the sustainable long term as it is built on major emotional fluctuations rather than set out frequent controlled enforcements that constantly keep in check your dietary intake.

However fasts should always be gradual renunciations of food until the next day you can have them. It is ok to stay today I will eat light and tomorrow I will eat heavy, however make sure they are not the case of major fluctuations where you only are cancelling out from where you began, instead of making a positive progress throughout the week.

Another example sudden deprivation of the body's normal conditioning state, being the quality of bad food that your consistently ingest,from one extreme to another, would only gain impetus for your inclination to retrogress by reverting back to your bad eating lifestyle with excessive or bad food regimes, instead of realising a new horizon via incremental and frequent fasts and detoxes. This leads to unmanageable uncontrollable fluctuations in diet where we are not in control and therefore this extreme up and down only tire and exhaust your long term vision goals of achieving your desired weight loss objective and more susceptible to desperate measures by resorting to diet fad scams that do not address the underlining root cause of the problem. The missing link here is lifestyle-- outlook, behaviour attitude, perspective. It is the knowledge that having wine in a park with friends will have more potency than drinking alone in a 4 cornered room; it is the knowledge that exercise will help us to be more resistant to food poisoning episodes and will make that coffee more energetic. Whilst exercise within itself makes you more energetic. And where you will see having that piece of cake with coffee not only as senseless but undesirable, as your senses and appetites have been restored back to their natural and healthy levels. Therefore when your healthy, your perception of taste and preference is objectively better than you were with your passion for food which you no longer savoured the taste for anyway. So your appetiser would naturally be inclined to brushetta bread, not because it is healthy, but is now tasty.

Place and timing

Weight loss sounds temporary, once again it should be termed your new weight size.

Place and timing are also important as when we inhabit and frequent new circles and environment destinations, we generally resort to eating places predominant around that area.

Preparing your own lunch can go along way to prevent this diet driven by inhabitation routine. Especially when the place you have no choice to frequent, as it is the area around your work has very little good food to offer.

Controlling food preparation is an exercise of the intellect and a cultural lesson of food culture by being improved and staying in control of the food ingredients we ingest.

For example , Most restaurants use oils that contain transfatty acids of some sort. With obvious exceptions, make it a habit to ask and learn the different oils types. Many are often promoted as being healthy or sound like they actually come from flowers. Oh that is a big one!! you must do your own research regarding hydrogenated oils or trans fatty oils.

This already suggests the obvious and you will also save time, energy and money.

There are many oils like cottenseed and canola oil that are promoted as natural but are far from it. Simply eliminating those oils and sticking to almond coconut and especially extra virgin olive oil-- goes along way. Food knowledge is imperative-- remember becoming a little philosopher. Extra virgin is known as the best that provide essential fats to the body that are not fattening, if that makes sense. This shows to the what extent chemicals and processed foods actually drive fat. Remember there are good fats and bad fats.

Olive oil versus canola oil

Do not fall into the hype which is put out by traditional medicine regarding the promotion of canola oil (rapeseed) as superior due to its concentration of monounsaturated fatty acids. Olive oil is far superior and has been around for thousands of years. Canola oil is a relatively recent development and the original crops were unfit for human consumption due to their high content of a dangerous fatty acid called euric acid.

The beneficial health effects of olive oil are due to both its high content of monounsaturated fatty acids and its high content of antioxidative substances. Studies have shown that olive oil offers protection against heart disease by controlling LDL ("bad") cholesterol levels while raising HDL (the "good" cholesterol) levels. (1-3) No other naturally produced oil has as large an amount of monounsaturated as olive oil -mainly oleic acid.

Olive oil is very well tolerated by the stomach. In fact, olive oil's protective function has a beneficial effect on ulcers and gastritis. Olive oil activates the secretion of bile and pancreatic hormones much more naturally than prescribed drugs. Consequently, it lowers the incidence of gallstone formation.

Olive oil and heart disease

Studies have shown that people who consumed 25 milliliters (mL) - about 2 tablespoons - of virgin olive oil daily for 1 week showed less oxidation of LDL cholesterol and higher levels of antioxidant compounds, particularly phenols, in the blood.(4)

But while all types of olive oil are sources of monounsaturated fat, EXTRA VIRGIN olive oil, from the first pressing of the olives, contains higher levels of antioxidants, particularly vitamin E and phenols, because it is less processed.

The type of oil in food makes a good food become bad, it is to this extent making an effort on finding good oils matters for the well being of your diet regime.

Naturally not all diet books will address this fact as it is a political football where allot of money is dependent on the illusion. But I have established through reading articles in papers that it is the most single most contributing factor to obesity and being overweight today.

Olive oil onto salads is certainly not a fattening affair, they are lubricant for your cells and contain the right essential fatty acids necessary to lose bad fat and maintain health.

Termed as a fat, rather it becomes apparent that this particular fat,monunsaturated is essential to the proper functioning of the body and that if you do not have this balance, like diet fads do not promote, you cannot sustain a positive weight loss regime.

Food classifications have no help with this regard as food information disclaimers mention that the oils contain a high amount of the goods fats and so we associate any fats, as their classified , as all inherent bad fats. Be careful. It is the chemicals in the process of making the bad oils—that make it fattening! Chemicals and fat is a subject worthy on its own accord and too comprehensive to be thoroughly covered in this paper. But for your guidance and further reading. An essential.

In the Mediterranean, men and especially woman have plenty of this oil, being the consequence of a betterment of health and waist size than those that do without it.

It is an integral part to the Mediterranean diet , used in virtually everything. The olive oil containing uncomplex compounds that are easily digestible in contrast to other industrial oils used in fast food outlets

So olive oil is an essential food ingredient. Already the purchasing of a certain product will go a long way to improve our health by virtue of placement and availability equals developing and acquiring good habits. Stock this in your shelves as you will find that it is the single most applied ingredient in the Mediterranean diet regime. It is the basis for cooking, application onto salads and {of course the apple cider vinegar and balsamic vinegar are so powerful, you can count on having this enjoyable salad with crispy bread as one of those detoxs sessions you will do throughout the day. But it was not a detox but a whole lunch, well now you can how this lifestyle works when your eating and detoxing at the same time.

This is 30% of your efforts without trying, just by changing product.

If you like your meat or like to have plenty of carbohydrates, this is great, as long as you more often that not supplement that dish with a salad mixed in with extra virgin olive oil, balsamic vinegar, feta tomato onions and a little salt and lemon. What you will find is that this salad is the detox to the dish while at the same time conprises the main meal, this is the backbone and secret to eating with lifestyle rather than as to indulge or to diet.

When the salads neutralise the high acid content of the food, they also purge the food of its impurities through the stomach and digestive track and increase the efficiency of the body to process the good nutrients for the body to create renewed fresh blood and renewed oxygen through the arteries. Ladies and gentlemen this is the immune system's metabolism rate, the rate by which it efficiently restores the body to a pristine optimum state by enriching the enzymes in the stomach so that they are effectively transported {via metabolic pathways}to the cells . Carbohydrate catabolism is increased the efficiency rate by which the body breaks down carbohydrates into the body.

The amino acids or proteins are the building blocks of cells and so after digestion, the nutrients converted from the gut go into the reforming and maintaining of cellular structure in the body and the more effective it does this, the more likely after a heavy pizza or heavy meal to retain your weight the exact size as your metabolism rate is healthy and optimum.

Good lipids or fatty acids and carbohydrates are needed for this process so this shows from a simply biological bio chemical point of view how the high protein diet fad is pure folly.

Little detoxes everyday.

Here is an example of implementing philosophy to your eating regime, some say too much fluoride is bad for our brain cells and our health and so we have to take a huge leap into another area of interdisciplinary knowledge so to improve our daily health and regime interactions. eg. Check out the role of bernays had in public relations of the dental industry and after you read this you will be eating apples even when they are not very tasty.

But not here, this is food for thought for your own cultural and intellectual inquiry that produces a satisfaction of acquiring knowledge about ourselves and the nature of the world around us. That will no doubt motivate us to be ever more vigilant of what we put into our mouths.

Knowledge of a food can induce a power and reason against the belly appetite to abstinence from it.

The brain and its conviction of belief is more powerful than our hunger pain urge in our belly.

Stay hungry if it will make you sick until you find a better food outlet to indulge in and never be afraid to ask questions or complain-- you are paying premium dollar for food today.

Say to yourself I have to eat at least one apple a day. This is a big movement, especially after a meal. This is the achievement of a little detox.

Why is it important to have fruit after a meal.

The ancient greeks always had a custom to serve fruit after a meal as they knew that it helped with the digestion process and cleaned the mouth. And co incidentally formed integrally as part of a natural detox regime

So often we see corporate knowledge promoted as real cultural knowledge.

More on marketing claims

Or in other words we see the packaging claims of a commercially driven product rather seeing the benefit of the actual natural product itself.

Commercially driven industry will not criticise the processed food industry, especially cheese and meat industry.

Real information is exchanged not via corporate to consumer, but through a caring person to another caring person in the community who has no inherent ulterior motive but the love and sympatheia of exchange of knowledge of learning and the thing that drives us all is empathy through compassion inherit in our natural communal nature and treatment of one another. In an age of globalisation this safety net mitigation is next to non existent and there are more stupid, selfish people than ever in a society that worships the individual and the concepts of instant convenience and self gratification.

The natural in build security mechanisms of community that bind and hold community have been demolished to the roads of globalisation where product value is pushed according to profit incentive rather than real value health incentive. You have to discern the difference.

We can have trust through the testimony of experience through the living daily people around us, who have tried and tested and have discerned and have the truthful motive to guide. This is the construct to a better society. There are still those few amongst us who care to mention that cold and flu tablets are unnecessary.

KIWI: Tiny but mighty, and a good source of potassium, magnesium, vitamin E & fiber. Its vitamin C content is twice that of an orange!

AN APPLE a day keeps the doctor away? Although an apple has a low vitamin C content, it has antioxidants & flavonoids which enhances the activity of vitamin C, thereby helping to lower the risk of colon cancer, heart attack & stroke.

STRAWBERRY: Protective Fruit. Strawberries have the highest total antioxidant power among major fruits & protect the body from cancer-causing, blood vessel-clogging free radicals.

EATING 2 - 4 ORANGES oranges a day may help keep colds away, lower cholesterol, prevent & dissolve kidney stones, and reduce the risk of colon cancer.

WATERMELON: Coolest thirst quencher. Composed of 92% water, it is also packed with a giant dose of glutathione, which helps boost our immune system. Also a key source of lycopene, the cancer-fighting oxidant. Also found in watermelon: Vitamin C & Potassium..

GUAVA & PAPAYA: Top awards for vitamin C. They are the clear winners for their high vitamin C content. Guava is also rich in fiber, which helps prevent constipation. Papaya is rich in carotene, good for your eyes..

Drinking Cold water after a meal = Cancer!

There is your nice flat stomach in the morning when the fruit has neutralised all the bad acid and harmful bacteria before it is distributed into your blood.

This obviously brings maximum metabolism to your body as your system breaks down fat so efficiently when you eat fruit everyday, that that cake you ate would not make any difference to how you feel as it would break it down and digest it quicker than you can imagine.

The universal understanding is that we all have the same experiences in life is what drives empathy and change. It is the only thing that makes us function, as cheesy as it sounds— love.. saying please and thankyou striking a conversation and making and maintaining friends, these days is an art within itself that has testified its benefits from generation to generation.

This is in essence what the mediterranean diet encompasses, the product of a community tradition in communion with nature and its seasons that produces true happiness, true health and true beauty. Technology can never overcome nature and the whole scientific progress thing is a pseudo religion within itself built on the medieval tenet that man can control nature. We are witnessing this frightening reality now with genetically altered crops etc.

Back to detox

Eating fruit after a meal is like virtually a little detox.

When we eat an apple, we acquire pleasure not just from the taste, but from the idea that we are cleaning our body and maintaining and sustaining the health of our teeth which its state is always an indication of our health anyway. I cannot emphasise this more!!!

4. Curb all sorts of cancers

Scientists from the American Association for Cancer Research, among others, agree that the consumption of flavonol-rich apples could help reduce your risk of developing pancreatic cancer by up to 23 per cent. Researchers at Cornell University have identified several compounds— triterpenoids—in apple peel that have potent anti-growth activities against cancer cells in the liver, colon and breast. Their earlier research found that extracts from whole apples can reduce the number and size of mammary tumours in rats. Meanwhile, the National Cancer Institute in the U.S. has recommended a high fibre intake to reduce the risk of colorectal cancer.

Detoxify your liver

We're constantly consuming toxins, whether it is from drinks or food, and your liver is responsible for clearing these toxins out of your body. Many doctors are skeptical of fad detox diets, saying they have the potential to do more harm than good. Luckily, one of the best—and easiest—things you can eat to help detoxify your liver is fruits—like apples.

Boost your immune system

Red apples contain an antioxidant called quercetin. Recent studies have found that quercetin can help boost and fortify your immune system, especially when you're stressed out.

One apple has just 95 calories, making it the perfect low calorie snack when a craving strikes. With zero fat & cholesterol, and very little sodium you can see why an apple a day has become so popular. Although not as high in fiber as some other foods, the high fiber count in apples gives them much of their fat-burning properties.

Many crucial vitamins can be found in relatively large numbers in just one apples, including vitamins C, K and B6. These vitamins are important for normal human functioning that promotes good health, which we know has a positive effect on fat burning.

Potassium is yet another nutrient that increases the health benefits of apples, with 195 mg found inside a medium apple.

Health Benefits of Apples

Because apples have long been considered a food that promotes good health, more research has been done to find out just how beneficial apples are to ideal health.

There are many antioxidants in apples that block absorption of harmful free radicals that can age you prematurely and cause disease. The polyphenols responsible for the antioxidant benefits of apples also help reduce artery clogging than can lead to heart health problems. These same anti-inflammatory properties are why apples help reduce asthma-related swelling.

The fiber content also improves the heart health benefits of apples, which has been known to reduce bad cholesterol. By literally eating "an apple a day," you can reduce the risk of many cardiovascular problems that include heart disease and stroke.

New research indicates that apples have an amazing ability to fight several types of cancer, but the lung cancer results have been especially promising.

I could not imagine a more effective way to detox that enjoyable dinner or lunch, especially if it was junk food and you get that fatty feeling in your stomach.
Eating applies with filtered water will almost certainly take your body back to square one and if you still feel bloated, then accustome your day, have another apple and more fruit and a light salad for lunch until your square one. Now the effort you made the get rid of that fatty lunch or dinner made you do all that work and so your less inclined to eat that bad take out again especially if it also made you sick as they usually also do.

Toothpaste only masks the symptoms as like certain pharma drugs and their action in masking disease rather than solving the root cause of the problem is apparent.
Even though there is an importance of cleaning your teeth, this is not an excuse to avoid having fruit.
This is why god made fruit is to restore the digestive bacteria state back to its prime original condition and then digestion will be more effective in cleansing all the toxins from the body.
Notice when you eat cheddar like cheese that the breathe stays even after eating an apple, showing that the breathe is also a great marker of health and we should be accustomed and stay in touch with this as a bearing and compass to the road of a more healthy lifestyle change success. Self reflection self observation.
The liver's function in cleaning toxins is heightens in a more alkaline state body.
Just a little about the immune system, that has been confirmed and corroborated by many leading scientists is that when the body has a acidic alkaline level brought on by unhealthy eating and lifestyle, then the body is more prone and susceptible to disease and when the body has a more positive alkaline level, brought on by good living and habualising eating nutritional beneficial foods, then disease and susceptibility is decreased and immunity function restored, and as metabolism resistant indicator maintained.
Metabolism and immunity are intrinsically linked. Meaning health and diet are intrinsically linked. So no more saying that girl is genetically got a great immune metabolism==no she is clean and healthy and has a correct outlook to life, observing and interplaying the variables of her lifestyle diet to the desired effect that is highly regularised as manifested through her good diet habits and inclinations.
So you cannot have a body without actually being healthy, you cannot cheat nature, unless the insurance protected diet fad products have something to say about that as they don't want to offend and say it is your fault, buy say it is natures.

So this is why today in order to be fate free, it means to be healthy and let me state it—being a philosopher who can control and mitigate his own balance and destiny according to the rhythms of the universe.

We cannot be blindly trusting and ignorant of the available food around us.

Even though we cannot get rid of all the hormones additive and pesticides they put into our food which unfortunately is another story of the role of chemicals in storing fat in the body and is the major reason for cellulite , we can compensate for this by the use of herbs, garlics and gingers in our bean salads and the spring onions and by living a frugal vigilant life with plenty of active engagements with friends and plenty of exercise—preferable outdoor exercise tennis or soccer.. that is also stimulating to the mind as it encompasses the social element that is vitally as important as the activity. I never understood blind obedient to exercise in the gym-- although it has its rightful place.

Of course garlics and chilis are fat burning, cleaning your blood on your own is something no doctor can ever compare. And we have shown that apples are also.

Onions and the Fat Burning Benefits
Onions, along with some of the other onion-family foods, help stimulate weight loss due to their natural richness of chromium. Chromium is an essential nutrient that improves the efficiency of insulin in the blood stream. With a more stable insulin release pattern, the body is able to maintain blood sugar levels, leading to more stable feelings of energy and stamina. While enhanced energy is certainly a perk, the greater benefit of stable energy and sugar levels is derived from the body's ability to abstain from food cravings and hunger. With stable energy and sugar levels, the body is less likely to send out hunger pains, as oftentimes the body will crave sugary and unhealthy foods in order to experience a short-term energy fix. If individuals consume foods that lead to an overproduction of insulin, the body encounters a low-energy crash and continues down the food-craving hunger pathway. Providing the body with chromium, onions help consumers feel more energized and fuller for longer periods of time, allowing consumers to comfortably restrict their caloric intake as they burn off stored fat to boost the body's functioning.

So their is no secret to weight loss, it is simply about maintaining metabolism within the body and so when everything is functioning properly then your digestive systems ability to empty out the desirables is increased, at the same time, the body ability to energize the body with nutrients is compounded and increased. This process with onions touted as a miracle cure will do just that. But shallots and garlics and other spicy food will do the same. It is about co ordinating them in food dishes which bring more taste with your food and are the little detox restorer you need for the body to maintain a fat free lifestyle.

Fat Burning Onions
With only 35 calories in each half cup of onions, this flavorful vegetable can be added to many savory foods and dishes.

At the same time, these spicy ingredients clean your blood so you can see fat burning and cleaning are intrinsically linked and cannot be separated. Diet fads separate the two and therefore blow out of context what true and lasting weight loss actually is.

Is this why generally Asian people are never overweight because of all these spices and herbs?? It is obvious a recycled notion about the excessive food consumption in the western world and how these diets have seen the greatest incidence of lifestyle caused diseases , the world has ever seen. Lifestyle meaning they are preventable and up to us to change our lifestyle and perspective if not for your weight then at least for your health.

Appreciating these foods means acquiring an appreciation for food culture and cuisine.

It also demands a respect for nature the knowledge and understanding that it is only through nature that we can be sure to stay connected to ourselves and stay connected with our health.

This does not mean eating raw foods, unless your really sick, but using natural foods from groceries in the use of food recipes . meaning that you have to appreciate and participate in food culture and become a little chef. Unfortunately we are caught up with expecting and demanding pre packaged food for our convenience and because of our little time, well then maybe in this day and age of an impending economic crisis we are now chastised and forced to change our diets by spending less at take outs and investing more time in our cooking and our health.

Do not follow every recipe that says to apply butter, put olive oil instead. Be smart!

Eating an apple is like a check, a self reflection and a opportunity to avoid those dentists who you cannot always trust with your teeth.

I started eating an apple a day more because I was scared that the condition of my teeth would make me suffer the gloom of an dentist appointment, but I learnt it is in this way, god and nature gets us to even maintain our health, sometimes out of fear, and if weight gain is your fear, compensation and prudence is in order cause by this way we also save our heath. So weight measurement can be a good gauge or meter to your health , but is not the only one. Sometimes the fear of getting fat can do allot to maintain our health. We just need to channel this according to the right actions and responses and never resort to excessive purging actions rather make it a learning experience to do it better the next time. Think of that time of your bloat after a crappy meal as a period of chastisement whereby you are mentally and physically and emotionally building resistance and strength to slowly change your habits and inclination. It is only through life and experience of life that we make changes. Only through failure do we find success. Remember being weak is not bad.

When we learn about these dynamics of the body and why we respond as we do, then we do allot to integrate our eating habits with our lifestyles. Perhaps we eat more when we are all inactive.

Definitely this is not an perception but a real objective realisation. Emotional binge eating and boredom are closely aligned and telling. Food is replacing a natural desire to participate in activity and we only eat food to try to compensate for this inadequacy in our lives--- it is this interactive multifaceted dimensional thinking we always should engage in because there is nothing like living a good and healthy lifestyle and avoiding laziness. So we need to replace this excessive food we eat with more occupation and activity that naturally takes our mind off eating. When we exercise and eat well during the day – it is always rewarding to see the results to our body. I guess on a superficial level this can be motivating and beneficial. There is nothing wrong with wanting to look good. As a matter of fact this is the central issue to this ebook. But we should never obsess about and resort to cosmetic surgery. God made you beautiful as you are and you ought to look after yourself and continue looking good cause there are many people out their much more unfortunate than we are.

So the day can be comprised of a series of chastisements and rewards that can characterise and build the patterns of our new lifestyle.

Fact—imported garlic is irradiated and bleached and gassed so use organic Australian garlic or garlic from your regional town.. cannot emphasise this more.

Garlic like olive oil, like apple cider vinegar should all be main ingredients to most of your lunch dishes do a google search of their health benefits and you will see how if these foods were packaged in glossy packaging show casting all these benefits, we would in fact spend more money on them than what they are listed for. It is these foods that allow us the fall out propensity to eat junk every now and then, because the amount of nutrients and anti oxidants in these foods overwhelm any bad snack you eat in the day and so you remain after the day in the positive. When we have this room to fall out or eat junk, they give us a sense of space by which we can more freely participate in our routine lifestyle without the unnecessary pressure and restraints/restrictions of diet fads and so as a result we have the incentive and impetus to do better as we are encouraged and rewarded for our actions.

Remember I am here to inform you that you will not only improve your health and weight, but prevent illness through knowledge of being informed.

Many of these foods are known to prevent cancer by maintaining the immune system.

So it is not to separate medicine with food , they are one,but make it a lifestyle where you are in control. Physically ,mentally and spiritually. Love god and love life, remember there is purpose in life and god has made life for us to participate and to struggle in his name the lord jesus christ.

When we get sick we ought to not always try to mask the problem with the use of pharmaceuticals, but sometimes and allot of the time we have to find the cause of the problem cause therein lies the true cure.

Otherwise we may have to rely unnecessarily on drugs which are known to build fat by destabilising the balance of our holistic field and total body health state and have shown in numerous cases to do make you more sick than the original disease you were treated in the first place.

Hippocrates mentions that the onset of disease occurs when the consumption of food exceeds the amount of exercise you engage, as the excess fuel changes your original composition and then your body signals an imbalance in the body that it alerts so that you may change a behaviour. Hippocrates saw a conflict between money and medicine and always advocates a philosophical approach to medicine, that is a philanthropic approach whereby the individual constitution of the person was analysed and then treated, not like today where people are generically treated without reason, cause or exploring the nature of the disease.

The 3 nutrients are solid food, drink and pneuma or air and the blanaced proportion intake of these are necessary to keep the bodies constitution in a primo state.

So is their a time when you drank when you should have walked on the beach and soaked in the sun? Would this in fact acted as a food of replenishment within itself?

Is their a time when you drank and you were really hungry, foolishly trying to cheat nature and loss unnaturally those extra kilos without in consultation with the bigger picture?

Is their a time, most importantly when you ate and you were really hungry?

These 3 states have to self criticised and evaluated as when you restore your functioning senses and constitution, your natural appetite will be restored and you will be eating and drinking at the right times and taking in air walking or jogging or exercising at the right times too. Therefore as a result of this balance being restored, your stomach size will be reduced and you will loss weight in accordance to a maintainable lifestyle addressed from a holistic point of view. Look at it as if you were solving all your health ,beauty and weight issues in one. Aren't we in the days of packages whereby we are more enticed by a product if it offers more things in the one package? So too you should commit to your health through self observation and reflection. This is the art of philosophy.

The ancient greeks never separated philosophy from engineering, from medicine, from mathematics, from architecture. If a structure or theory did not address or solve to better the existence of man is a philanthropic setting then it was deemed unproductive.

Today unproductive is anything that does not make incredible profits for companies, usually at the expense of people's healths. So you must be empowered and wear your toga so to speak.

So eating excessively is a sort of sickness that needs to be corrected according to these 3 templates. A part cannot be addressed without the whole as the part is essentially a function and connection to the whole whereby if the part was treated merely for its own sake, the whole would be deprived and the set change desired of your action would not occur.

When you build up a strong food lifestyle regime with a series of recipes and regimes coupled with exercise etc, you become accustomed to listening to your body, what makes you feel sick and what makes you feel good and healthy, by keeping a material{making a note in diary for example} of what actions/behaviours and particular foods you had in one day and describing how you reacted to them. This will help us improve and formulate our regime the next day and preserving effective habits for the next day and it keeps us in control of our health. Learn about true medicine and true health. This ebook is not about politics in medicine but merely encourages you to adopt the right lenses by which to view and engage the world so you are more informed and better off.

Hippocrates notes the best physician is thy self and these and many more principles find relevance still in this time in live in.

By doing this, you stay in tune with the holistic wisdom and knowledge that most diseases today are caused by our lifestyle and by the pollution in our environment despite the genetic origin of disease mongers who profit from pseudo medical theories that our genes somehow contribute to disease without emphasizing the role of the lifestyle and environment have on our health.

When we continuously eat bad food, this compromises our immune system and the proper theory of medicine dictates that when we learn to be our own physician of our own bodies by consciously staying in touch with eating good foods, we learn how to prescribe ourselves an antidote to our ill health when we become sick because we know instinctively that our sickness was activated by lack of exercise or bad thinking processes and lifestyle stress and eating habits. We innately learn that health is the natural state of the body, that we need to maintain.

So we simply employ corrective measures through the eating habits that we have already presumably integrated into our lifestyle. setting the Right of the wrong and replenishing the deficiency or the excess and restoring the natural constitution and homeostasis of mankind to the original state.

The total person encompasses the mental emotional and spiritual faculties and when we live a clean and healthy lifestyle, {not just with the food we eat}, then we maintain our health for the long term wholesome good.

So if you find yourself always in the house, some days it is ok to stay home than to make plans with friends. Sometimes an occasion with friends is exercise in itself. Walking reflecting, inspiring, contemplating stimulating the senses and infusing all that vital hippocrates pnuema for your cardiovascular system. The cool air drawing deep in the night is the best because the trees have metabolised allot of the days pollution by that point and there is no more pollution of the streets. To draw this air is imperative to your health no matter how much you exercise.

When we are over worked, maybe excessive exercising at the gym compounds your eating habits, as you are not getting enough rest. Maybe we are eating too much meat. Do a quick google on the subject. Google is a powerful database which will source you information that corroborates the facts for your comfort. You will notice a consensus of ideas from varying resources that support the truth. Remember public scrutiny paves its own channel of truth free from the distortions of the commercial media saturating a particular theory of a product to the minds of the masses whereby we sponge our ideas not from real communicative information through the communion of community but by corporations that only owe their allegiance to their stock holders.-.

why do we watch so much tv?

Real rest should be reflective, or inspiration like walking the beach at night gazing into the moon, or spending time alone reading or preferably researching food medicine.

Rest is easing the mind and the body for renewal and rejuvenation it is a recreation, like a day at the beach or a visitation to a friend, not watching TVs.

So get a diary and plan your week.

Everything is interrelated.

When we live out of balance, our bodies produces signals of stress and it is important to remember that the throat coughs because it is the natural healing mechanism of the body that is activated when the person is suffering an aliment so the immune system of the person produces a cough to get rid of the ailment in the throat. This is your natural internal guide within you.

So therefore the role of medicine is to nurture and this symptomal process until the body goes back to its original prime healthy state.

All diseases have a root and a cause. But it is important to know that is not always the food we eat, but sometimes our attitude and outlook in life and so this is another realm altogether.

Drugs simply mask symptoms and may have temporary benefits but because they do not address the root cause of the problem, they do not cure the person, nor do the pharma drugs claim to do so anyway as the word cure is repugnant and abhorrent in professional medical /pharmaceutical circles. A doctor for example will not mention and admit that the cheese your eating is making you feel sick. It is out of his periphery.

When you eat industrial sludge commercial cheese ,for example you will notice after affects, like sticky perspiration, slight heaviness, bloated stomach and feeling of general ill health.

For an average healthy person, the metabolism of a person may take 2-5 hours to get rid of these effects and this is without medicinal food, but just rest. So you inadvertently crowd up and exhaust your metabolism for the other more beneficial foods we may consume.

As a result your respiratory metabolism is switching to safe mode, rather than unobstructively drawing in the vital energy from the air for your constitution.

However for a unhealthy person that regularly has bad food, that is subsequently affecting his mental and mood states, it would take longer for his metabolism to get rid of the affects as his immune system is in a unhealthy low state and be more susceptible to opportunistic infections like the common cold and then if left unchanged chronic illness may eventuate.

Exercising.

Unfortunately most people associate exercise as something you periodical take out away from your routine and excessively run on tread mill and get home and not feel so guilty about that binge latter on. We see it as separate to the routine of our lifestyle. But when we work we are burning calories, when we walk we are exercising and when we play soccer we are also exercising even though it does not feel like it because the added benefit to mental stimulating sports is that it is engaged in a social setting so therefore you getting 2 benefits for one. One is the mental pneuma stimulation, the vital air of social ability a medicine within itself that mandates the common phrase, love is the cure. And the other is the obvious physical exertion and pressure that builds resistance,endurance and strength to your body; both these compliment each other whereby exercise now becomes an enjoyable leisure and social occasion rather than a prolonged delayed and boring one watching the kilometre clock on the treadmill in front of TVs. In the gym. The vital air component makes the gym cardio expereince less effective and efficient because it is usually indoors and the air cannot allow the body circulatory and cardio system to expand and contract in its optimum condition and the lack of oxygen makes for decreased capacity of recovery and less benefit per energy unit invested.

There is nothing wrong with going to a gym, for its obvious social benefits, being a club where you could meet people and be apart of something, however people get confined with the preoccupation with body image and over exercising as gyms do not usually offer diverse activities of exercising coupled with relaxation.

Many people damage their immune system and bodies by taking one extreme to another from an 8 hour shift straight to the gym is not the way to benefit your health in the long term.

Work balance is always possible, however one can demand more relaxation and flexibility in their working day. So the solution to exercise is that it ought to be a leisure slash past time slash exercise.

Having a walk and a long lunch break can be way more beneficial than excessive exercising after work and then having to crash out from your other hobbies, to only have to prepare tiredly for work the next day. Maintaining balance and energy is key.

Little exercises and stretches

Incorporating little exercises through the day brings about a lifestyle component to weight loss and lifestyle.

Crunches by your office desk, knee lift up to your stomach, reaching out and stretching the body. Invaluable!!!

Stretching is so underestimated, people forget to realise that muscle weight training is a form of stretches via regular interval contraction .

What is apparently most important when sitting down at work for large durations of the day is the ability and willingness to get up regularly, to walk around every hour, to stretch your back and do some knee crunches.

Your endurance and energy levels would improve at work and you will remain focused, and little exercises everyday is more sustainable and practical and more effective than preparing for a professional fitness marathon after work when your body has already burnt allot of energy just by sitting down. This is significant as walking and stretches in life balance will make you lose more weight and sustain in the long run that damaging your balance through over exercise. As we need fuel to loss weight and keep healthy. One can see a day cut out for work would demand rest as a more important recreational past time than exercise. Without balance –their is no health and without health there is no consistent weight size. Of course there are exemptions because a skinny person is not always a healthy person, the stress can manifest in other areas separate from weight gain.

Which brings me again to preoccupation with planning events, being busy makes you forget to eat sometimes, which can be put to good use , but in perspective as you do not want to make that an absolute consistent habit where we start ignoring genuine hunger or nutritional quest pains. Let pneuma or vital air energy be also your food. Learning is a cultural activity is also a sort of food or spiritual food more powerful than the blameless passion of food. Perhaps when you eat you need to be reading more and a coffee or black tea won't hurt.

Also being preoccupied, stressed and depressed may make you overeat, so be wary of these internal dynamics and observe their characteristics and adjust accordingly. This is the essence of self observation and reflection.

.Excess emotional binge eating compensates unnaturally the lack of physical exertion activity and pro activity in your daily regime.

Diversity of occupation and daily activity is essential and vital.

People become gym junkies and would sacrifice a day at the beach with their friends without them realising that not only will they form the ability to relax and attain a state of peace through the inspiration of the beach scenery through their participation with their senses to the smells, sights and sounds and be refreshed for the next week of work that lay ahead, they will also be consuming allot of energy simply be relaxing at the beach rather than excessively exercising and disturbing their metabolism cycles if they exercised on their own. They will also retain allot of vital energy where excessive exercise would have disturbed and the body to the point where it would need more energy in order for it to be restored and healed. So there is obviously a balance you need to gauge for yourself. Jogging once a week for example is more efficient per energy unit than 3 times a week. That is why the gym inadvertently promotes excess exercising save the social aspect of it

But then again there are also times when we need to be alone and away from friends where we self contemplate and reflect and this could very well be in the form of simply exercising on a tread mill in the gym--- we will all testify that light exercises are a way to alleviate stress and increase your propensity to relax and sustain a general sense of well being

So to lose weight a balance of rest and diet and occupation and mental stimulating exercise is in order. Or the balance proportional intake of solid food, drink and pneuma postulated by hippocrates.

Just like when people regularly miss eating lunch and dinner, they have no energy to lose weight and so they stay the same weight. Some people do not get enough of nutrition, enough of rest, or enough of exercise or enough of social event planning and when one is off balance we usually try to compensate this with over eating or over exercising or over binging etc.

usually fat people are in a state of respiratory and metabolic exhaustion whereby the body is so assaulted by bad living on every level that they need specific treatment pertaining to restoring their metabolic function. So they need to have more herbal teas and less coffees, no excessive exercising, but incrementally as they merely need to restore the 3 vital food intakes of hippocrates so they are restored to their correct functioning state by being in proportion each other other.

Excessively fat people are sick and their perception of food is tainted to the degree that the prospect of walking is abhorrent and repulsive to their senses as they are perfectly geared to this disharmony and disbalance

so food is not a fuel of enjoyment but a source of accumulation for accumulation sake, this is the essence of gluttony which is an illness to be treated because it starts in the psych y or the soul which has passions that are driving and controlling the person as like a parasite.

Unfortunately this is accumulated over time and so needs time to be corrected , even though the time it takes to be corrected can be much less than it took for the weight to accumulate throughout the years.

Don't suppress the body, the girls that have high metabolisms, enjoy their food more and know instinctively through listening to their weekly regime cycle that having a full stomach of food will be burnt off from their preoccupied weekly regime or rather a balanced weekly regime.

They see that day of rest or enjoying walk around town as a metabolistic health dieting exercise as this is integrally linked to good health promoting, weight losing style of lifestyle. This does not mean you go and exercise constantly.

She is the girl that always eats , never exercising or so she says, and still stays the same skinny weight, that is because she is probably choka block with weekly activity that is akin to exercise as she burns allot of energy doing this/. It also encompasses a healthy state of mind and also she may have regular fasts, which include abstinence for some of the day and also eating fruits that regularly clean the system.

But also they know when to sleep and relax with their own company and they do not disturb their metabolism via crazy drink binge sessions. They are more in touch with the natural cycles of their body and with the cycles of the universe and the seasons. But enjoying a couple of shots and one drink is all you need all night really!!! Do not rely on alcohol for a good night out, participate in conversation and socializing should always be in focus and expresses our inherent creative nature and urge as human being to commune with one another and to share. Alcohol has many chemicals and so the best alcohol that not only maximises our euphoric and relaxing states but can also be somewhat therapeutic is 2-3 cocktails a night. Cocktails with quality spirits which are properly processed and distilled and are quality drinks mixed with fresh juices which kick in the natural high tipsy feeling we are all trying to attain to unlock and unsettle the nerves from a tense week at work.

Remember allot of the effects of hang overs are exasperated by the chemicals inherent in them especially beer and especially the pre packaged alcohol drinks that have too much sugar. The spirits from my experience don't have this chemical latency effect. But don't take it from me try them and if they do not bloat and give you a good feeling then they may suit you. But once again it is about self observation and adaptation. Having the right drinks and the right quantities. Excessive alcohol binging that reek havoc to your body metabolic functioning even if they are the correct drinks.

Few effective exercise tips

While sitting down, do regular stretches, lift up arms and feel it in the buttocks and tummy.

While watching a movie on your bed , do not waste the opportunity to do knee crunches, knee to stomach then release fully straighten legs, this is addictive and you will see that your lazy state on your bed will turn to a energy filled period where you want to get up during the film, pausing and get those chips, preferably sunflower oil, but always always washed down with purified water.

Never stock up on chips, what is in your cupboard obviously determines your eating habits, so if you are going to watch a movie, go to the effort of going in your car to nearest petrol station and buy a semi sized chips, preferably plain as the chemicals in chips act as a extra fat building opportunity we can't always afford.

A realistic model is that we are human and sometimes we have cravings that we cannot help, but is all about mitigating and regularising these urges and preventing them from completely controlling us. We enjoy these sporadic naughty indulges more when we have a healthy lifestyle and not when it controls you. These are the little anomalies we can afford as our good habits cancel out the bad effects of these occasional binges. But we enjoy them more when they are on occasion and when you do it you are still eating and taking your time eating them allowing your body to digest and process them without a sudden accumulator effect. The capacity of water to clean the dirty oils in the body makes this binge a calculated one but still ravaging enjoyable, but sustainable.

You would be crazy to buy a soft drink with the chips, but if you have to, buy a small size or even those Italian chinotto drinks, that are more natural and very small.

Soft drinks are the major contributor to obesity, stamping out of your diet is the best thing to do. They function merely as occasional refreshments not as fundamental and primary fluids to quench your thirst. This is in accord to their proper place in your lifestyle and how they are meant to be taken as any half discerning person, will see the body sweating when excessive consumption has been made.

It is important to understand that soft drinks do not quench thirst and food companies research ways to make food addictive so they could sell more product. Nothing quenches your thirst more than water. Add stawberry, lemon and basil in there. Congratulations. Your well o n your way. Drinking this in the day will rejuvenate and clean you, build your energy and of course preserve your weight size or help you decrease it.

Keep in mind fresh juice as better than processed juices that are full of sugar and are still similar as having softdrinks.

Make a habit before going in to the shower do some star knee stretches, by repeat lift knees to stomach and down again while lifting up your arms doing it.

So important , this builds energy levels, metabolism endurance and resilience, a better general well being by making blood circulate around the body.

Remember it is important to have water after a coffee ,as coffee these days has allot of toxins and milk may end up a dead bio product that needs substantial digestion.

Hippocrates mentions that this bile can disturb the bodies constitution and block arteries.

One can almost say that excess fat in the body is dead matter building up clogging up the arteries, that is why excessively fat people need prescriptions of herbal medicine, or infused herbal teas to rebuild these damaged channels of veins and arteries so that vital air, oxygen and nutrition once again circulate to reinvigorate their metabolism and lymphatic system   t to properly flush out toxins through digestion and increase the ability and capacity of the body to retain good energy reserves to maintain optimum general immune system functioning. Now this explains in depth the real process of weight loss from a truly scientific and holistic point of view.

When we are accustomed to watch our alkaline levels so that our body does not become too acidic, then we are sure on our way to not just helping our weight, simply for the sustainable short term, but in the long term you solved the root problem of your lifestyle by self criticism/observation and genuine sincere convictions for incremental change by primarily focusing on health and lifestyle before superficially trying to unnaturally induce weight loss through diet fads, cold turkeys or other extreme and self violent means of induction. Remember this will aggravate rather than solve our health issues through our lifestyle.

When your blood terrain is clean from the accumulative effects of a good food, good drink good pneuma and general lifestyle, then your propensity for resisting disease grows, your propensity to keep a good weight is sustained and your general feeling of well being restored.

This shows that all your channel arteries are metabolising energy at its highest efficient rate by breaking down nutrients and the conversion of nutrients into oxygenated blood that perfectly restores your cardio system. Now the mystery metabolism is forever solved and your motivation to focus on your health as a way to improve your diet contextualised in your mind that will help you pave the way to mould a lifestyle routine that perfectly fits your particular constitution, environment and circumstance.

When our body is too acidic, then this is a marker for the state of our immune system, and we tend to be more over weight, more prone to disease and illness and bad mood levels.

Eating a fruit {antioxidant}after a coffee for example , is highly conscientious and understanding of the role of food is cleansing our body from the toxins that accumulate in our bodies. This is not a diet but a behaviour activity to a lifestyle situation.

Dieting presumes something separate from life and lifestyle which is the heart of solving your weight issues. The idea is to focus without anxiety and with patience becoming healthy, it is then weight loss will fall naturally as a consequence of this corrective directive you affected.

This is the balanced lifestyle, even though an apple is not the most tasteful of food, the ones that achieve their weight objectives, force themselves and discipline themselves to make sure they have one, because being in touch with themselves gives them the motivation to self clean themselves after eating something filling. It is about staying in touch with your self and listening to your body rhythms. It is recognising food not simply for pleasure but for life and for health . This is the essence of truly living the moment and truly living life which is appreciating life from a multifaceted point of view.

Perhaps they are aware that some coffee contains anxiety drugs and is spoilt and polluted in an age where food processing is on such a mass scale and in an age where food is a pure business commodity rather than a sacred substance made and stored for the proper nourishment of man, that sometimes you cannot tell truth from fiction unless of course you were aware and were vigilant-- I think it ought to be a duty to read the newspaper, it is therapeutic and makes us think about the world around us rather than being selfish and self consumed with our own desires and shortcomings.

Coffee is a food with obvious benefits and caffeine can be a drug that is good.

Coffee has many properties that are good for the heart, cardio system and our general well being.

Obviously when it becomes addictive this is an issue. This is where moderation interplays.

However coffee plays an important kick start metabolic role. Firstly psychologically focusing on drinking than eating and secondly its properties accelerate metabolism by increasing your energy rate. This effect can reflect your lifestyle whereby your looking for the lowest course of resistance to increase energy metabolism of your cell constitution whilst minimising the excessive energy reserves an impromptu lunch could create. So your more an air person focusing on drink would tend to placate the time you have food solids in its correct place. However many girls are unhealthy as they exaggerate this effect and you will see that their caffeine hits are no longer enough and they then have to resort to energy drinks which do damage to the heart and cardio system. It is best to eat a little toast with a coffee for example if you want to by pass lunch. But you need to compensate with carbohydrates at dinner to reinvigorate the lack of energy of your system in the day. Remember your body needs energy to loss weight because it is not about less food but re correcting the constitution of the body but proportioning the 3 in takes of food drink and pneuma.

When on the bed, do sit ups. These are form of stretches of resistance and highly beneficial.

On hot days, have smoothies, even though your use to coffee, your body much rather need hydration that a coffee hit.

What is also a consideration is when we have eaten allot for dinner and a few snacks and our stomach is full.

So if you are not hungry, don't have that cereal with the milk filled with all those calories and hormones.

Have a piece of fruit and go out.

However it is important that you do eat at least a sandwich latter on. Of course without butter.

If your still searching for food then you have not organised your time and engaged yourself in activity that will make you forget about food.

Vegetables are tasty and easy, even addictive

Having the 5 veges a day is not something difficult, in this day and age of gourmet that by combining food with herbs, makes you appreciate the use of vegetables in complementing flavours in your meats and seafoods.

As mentoned before and cannot stress more,Transfatty oils are abundant in the take out food market, that they on their own can constitute a sole contributing health threat, even when on they don't comprise a major element to your weekly eating regime, just one experience or visitation with one of these junk food places can significantly contribute to a deterioration of your immune system and spoil all the work you have done to maintain your immune system and you are also more likely to be food poisoned. Always make it a habit to ask about the food your ordering, although this is not always possible.

But once again a good lifestyle means greater tolerance and resistance to these sporadic unfortunate events of eating junk, so remember have confidence in your immune system when you feel sick after food to flush it out with lemon water or herbal tea for example. You will become stronger.

Canned food is bad partly for the reason that the salt levels are too much.

Here is a classic example of hippocrates principle whereby consumption must not exceed exercise or acquisition of vital air.

However hippocrates may not have foreseen a time where one serving of food could temporarily throw off your system to protection mode, for example excessive salt can inflame your heart sac or the protective barrier of muscle surrounding the heart and so if we are not exercising excessively in that given day it is best to avoid this canned food even though convenient because it is directing the body to cancel out the excess salt through exercise when it is impracticable and unreasonably to do so especially when it is simply to cancel out the effects of the intake of one food events. How uneconomical and burdensome is that.

Of course if you have a good immune system, the body will take time to metabolise these excessive salts and the inflammation process is a natural part to it at times. But it probably means that if you do have inflammation, then it is a key indicator to the general health of your basic constitution that one bad food event, even though the bad food event can trigger a metabolic renunciation like this one.

Filtered water can contribute as much as 25 % to your immune building efforts without effort to your new lifestyle diet routine.

Buy a filter with readily available water, make sure that the containers are composed of glass as the plastic can't strip into the water. Have softdrink occasionally, however to really quench your first always rely on cold filtered water.

Always make a habit of filling them with filtered water and putting them in the fridge.

If you want some taste or you 'd like to clean the water a little more, put rosemary, strawberry , mint and lemon in the water. Olive oil and especially filtered water is the lubricant and medium the body uses to transmit signals, to break down chemicals for the efficiency of your metabolism.

This is so important that you hydrate yourself in the summer with water, rather than in vain try to fill your thirst up with sugar topped softdrinks that bloat your stomach.

As a beverage they are great to have around, but do not store them unnecessarily and have them just laying in the fridge waiting for you to drink them.

Eating with our emotional states

An important thing to consider and is part of this whole idea of keeping in context and perspective, is when we neglect an aspect of our lives, when we are bored, imbalanced, taking too much prescription drugs without identifying the cause or looking after our bodies in harmony and maintenance, most diets, as well intentioned, are in vein and will be quickly categorised as instant diet fads that make you shoot up and down without keeping the pounds off permanently As they do not address the underlining issue and cause that is inextricably stemmed in lifestyle diet and exercise.

when you don't embrace your new lifestyle by learning to habitualise it and beginning to feel comfortable with it,this will change your weight without effort instantaneously before your eyes. All your newly acquired healthy activities are integrated into your new lifestyle and so it is no longer unattainable to reach your weight goals as their already a living breathing reality within the context of your new lifestyle change. This is of paramount importance because it is fad diets that add pressure to our lives and as a result we crash and have to begin again. A horrible reciprocally damaging to us psychologically to rebuilt impetus and courage again.

Because a correct lifestyle is without excessive effort, but a well planned day where you are self monitoring your actions, through incremental improvement patterns of behaviour and anticipating how to moderate and compensate to ensure that after the course of the day you have achieved balance and homeostasis. Or restore your body to its natural harmonic vibrating state which is health. Doctors will make you believe that the body is geared to sickness but this is medieval folly. This is another story.

Make sure your routine is spontaneous and rhythmic not robotic. The central theme is enjoyment throughout the day and that food plays the role to compliment it.

You know that good food is a happy mood stabiliser and so correct eating will make you enjoy the day better. Better at articulating your thoughts with your friends, greater feelings of optimism and a day of better general performance throughout the day. This is the essence of living and filling up your day to its maximum potential. This is what characterises the good day.

No matter what we do, we must always look to exercise everyday as much as we can and there are no short cuts. However the reason this becomes easy is because we learn how it makes us feel better, look better and feel healthier especially when we exercise to play where we are exercising but really playing. Forgetting about the stop watch, how many calories you have lost because it was not an obligatory experience but an enjoyable one. Play basketball with friends, play tennis or soccer. Playing in groups is paramount as you attain more benefit for your exercise. Do this now! You may also meet some beautiful people.

But this is not excessively exercising at the gym, but a little bit of stretches in the morning, some skipping before you go into the shower for the morning. This can be as little as 15 minutes. This cannot be emphasised more. Get into a club enjoy your exercise not as work but as a leisurely activity and as a form of real rest and play not added burden.

By skipping breakfast and just having an apple does allot for the metabolism. Because you had a nice full meal the night before or you binged out. But if not eat a couple of toasts fat free italian style bread preferably gluten free and with no butter, and never be afraid of having eggs for breakfast as they nutritious.

So eating correctly and being full is a different type of full feeling in the stomach than if you had just eaten junk food. remember this. The junk food full is not really full but as a fool you will still want to eat more because your body still craves for food as it has not been replenished nutritionally.

Smaller portions can train a smaller stomach. It takes approximately 5 minutes after eating for the hunger pains to leave, so it is not always good idea to eat to hearts content but remember that when your body is trained to eat well, the occasional over eating will easily be adapted by the body and would not make a difference to your health and diet.

You'd be silly to not eat bread with a salad, you need to be content and happy from eating. Remember the body constitution in balance proportion is the solution not avoiding certain foods that are really nutritious and invaluable to your general health and then your subsequent improved waist line. So once again eggs are in. what a great source of protein. The building blocks of your cells. With an improved lifestyle you can still enjoy your food.

Every meal should have some salad.

Now you may be used to chips and fish or meat and rice, but without salad, not only are you missing out the health benefits, you are missing a sense of food cuisine and culture by missing out on the taste of the food. This is indispensable.

Salad essentials

Onions, tomato, paisley, lettuce and tomato with olive oil, balsamic vinegar.

Eat shallot with tomatoes a little bit of bread and olives—this is a little tonic before you hit out to town.

This tastes fantastic and when people do not learn to acquire taste for these foods, then they could not be healthy even when they are skinny, because some people are really skinny and keep it that way by suppression or by excessive binging then excessive fasting in response.

Often woman are besieged with the prospect of that by eating at take outs or some other fast food, latter they will decide not to eat latter to compensate that.

One has to understand that chemicals in food are one of the major contributors of weight gain, not the food itself.

When you think of a burger, It is meat and a bun.

If it was a quality patty which is 100 % thigh meat or something like that, with the salad in the bun, it is a good meal, but when the meat is a product of the whole animal being squashed, your body is suddenly immersed with the daunting prospect of working itself overtime to clean itself up.i believe meat should be avoided because of all the hormones and antibiotics and other chemicals they use in its production. It is known that after eating meat your blood ph level for the first 2 hours could equal to that of a cancer patient. If you must better a chicken burger and one that is preferably grilled, better yet have salmon this would replace the meat eating desire feeling

It is best to determine a habit not to eat at fast food chains often.

But make it a habit that if you do fall, then when you have that tummy ache or you are bloated, let that be the motivation to say to oneself not to eat there for at least 3 months, until you fall again and then maybe make a resolution not to go for 6 months or never at all. This can be allowable and feasible within a lifestyle pattern that we still successfully reduce your weight and improve your health for the long term.

There are many documentaries that can turn you off from meat products, which stay in your belly for prolonged durations of time and is hard for the body to digest it. It is not just the meat but the hormones and chemicals in the meat.

It is not about scaremongering but about being informed as a philosopher and never to think, I am going to starve myself on Saturday so I look better and fit into that incredible dress/.

It is important that you always eat 3 meals in the day or even 4-5 meals in small portions.

Sometimes missing lunch breakfast every now and then is ok.

Cause it can fit into a lifestyle where you are so much enjoying or preoccupied with something you forget to eat. But please never make it a habit.

Discipline is sometimes not enough, but being informed about eating out and paying extra for sub standard foods and oils, can be motivation enough to starve it off until you reach home.

It is fine that from time to time you want to enjoy on spontaneity from eating , however not if it makes you sick.

But better you pack lunch, conserving money and resources and those kilos. These are the little logical steps you can employ in between meals.

Replacing snacks for more healthy alternatives.

Gelato instead of ice cream. But ice cream is ok.

A toast instead of banana bread.

Coffee without much milk. And with water.

Cut donuts out all together and substitute it for toast and jam.

Fruit after a bad meal or any meal will always clean your body to restore it normal functioning. Take an apple before work.

Adding onions and shallots in your fred eggs and some pasley and tomato.

98% fat free bread, rather than standard.

Buying smaller chips instead on bulking on larger chips.

Keep cupboards without junk. I wll say it again. Not even biscuits, these are trans fatty compounds hard for the body to digest. Especially if your addicted but if you know you have them irregularly anyway in your pre existing regime , buy simple arnotts, nice biscuits without the chocolaty high compound stuff. But coffee breaks – need only a simple toast, no cake.

Force yourself if hungry at night – to eat something and then have camomile tea before sleep with fruit when you wake up. Especially when you have been feeling sick or had too much to drink over the weekend.

When binged out at night, drink plenty of water and have some fruit in the morning.

This is lifestyle eating. Eating, detoxification and self cleaning and it is all without effort as long as you train yourself that way.

 let it be it a motivation for the health of your teeth to keep that dentist away by eating that fruit regularly everyday. Toothpaste merely masks bad breathe, remember your mouth terrain is a reflection of what you eat and your mouth is a reflection of the state of your body terrain or environment.

Let this be a motivation and sometimes fear is the best deterrent when it is discovered what all those lollies and sugar sweets are doing to your teeth.

Buy mixed bags of nuts and dried fruit and dried bananas, you don't have to have them all the time as a snack food or vege out, but just incorporating them in your schedule, you will create some balance, even when you fall from time to time and have chips and chocolates.

It is easy for us to develop sore teeth these days from all the processed food we eat.

If you recall after having cheddar cheese, how your breathe stinks, almost no matter what cleansing type fruit meal you have, it is still present. This shows that the mouth is a reflection of the current state of our heath and so we can use it as a gauge.

Toothpaste and mints simply disguise the smell and the methol does to an extend have some cleaning effect, but cleaning teeth at night is no justification for you not to eat that fruit after a meal.

This is imperative to good health. Acquiring the taste of fruit , but most importantly acquiring the consciousness of the condition of your mouth after you've eaten meat, cheese or coffee.

Harness the foresight to smell your own breathe and recognise that this is now in your stomach and by altering the breathe of your mouth with a piece of fruit, you are altering the chemistry of your body by neutralising your acid levels so your body is restored to its healthy alkaline state. This is a perfect example of self reflection and living a vibrant healthy life.

This proper restoration of the alkaline state of your body is that pervasive metabolism that your friend always bragged that she was born with it.

Remember this gene theory of disease and predisposition to disease by genes and predisposition to having a worse off metabolism is highly contentious so do your own research.

When your lazy and not preoccupied we compensate this by eating more.

Being active and occupied will almost always burn kills without the effort of doing so.

Recreational exercise like swimming takes allot of energy to pack, to drive to organise, swim and then shower and return home. And the breeze remains in your mind unlike the gym.

Activity is not confined to the physical or extreme exertive exercise, remember a well planned out day conducting business routine or creative occupation of some sort , will make you lose so many calories before any preconceived consciousness of doing so. This is the essence of the lifestyle and this is where the propensity lies for us to eat more of what we like and enjoy our food , instead of it being a weight and burden that is unbearable and unworkable.

You will do allot for your health by just maintaining your health by staying extra vigilant to recognising the role of medicinal foods have in maintaining our health. Get a natural therapy encyclopaedia. Buy a essential oil burner, become acquainted with herbs and the best fat burners known to man. Onions, garlics and chili.

It therefore becomes an exercise of constant spontaneous adaptation For example when you have tomato and cucumber olive platter with bread, incorporate some Australian garlic. This only increases the taste, but also helps with your current sickness.

The problem is once you have garlic with tomato and cucumber with oregano and herbs, olive oil and basil a natural antioxidant anti inflammatory, then you will probably not go back, because the mix of these foods in your mouth are just exquisite. Once you restore your natural food tasting faculties through incremental diligence and reconditioning your habits towards the original state, you will realise you will be more happier and not feel propelled to go back to your old lifestyle. It is not about artificially building new habits, but restoring yourself, your communion with nature and restoring the balance in your life. There is no addiction or passion or habit here, but life as meant to be experienced all in moderation and variety. Most importantly without feeling that you are doing so because you will see the benefits gained from a holistic point of view.

If you do not like the taste, start liking the taste.

There is no distinction between medicine, health and dieting, as they inherently form the lifestyle of our daily lives. This is paramount and it is up for all of us to discover their own path of awareness and get out of the fat and non fat dialectic way of thinking. This is unhealthy for the mind as it does not address the underlining cause which is centred in lifestyle.

When the body becomes diseased it is really a signal the body transmits that there is an imbalance in the body and that you need to do something to correct it.

This signal is usually labelled as a disease, however when one views this process from a thorougher scientific point of view, they will realise that this so called disease is really the body's attempt to restore itself to its natural original condition.

This is done through the immune system. A great book to read and I recommend is pasteur's germ theory exposed. Understand true medicine therefore understand true health from the masters.

Good products to get you to save money and maintain your healthy lifestyle.

Projection of vegetables in media made you see vegetables as a bother, I think It is generally understood now that the role of vegetables is to compliment the main course with flavour while adding health benefits to the dish. A win win situation as nature intended.

Initial effort is in order to change your habits and sometimes you need to sacrifice as the lifestyle mantra encompasses the idea that attaining the highest value from your day.

Once your initial exposure to the obstacle of fighting yourself away from a certain food is over, all other subsequent exposures will become gradually easier. This is written down as behavioural theory is psychology. Or better described as when we are exposed to our fears, our bodies learn slowly and incrementally to get used to this change.

Maintaining a lifestyle is all about this. Sometimes keeping checks and balances, sometimes compensating, but always rhythmic harmonic and overall is easy given the opportunity cost involved, being the value and priority of your health and your looks.

Generally eating a variety of foods is the way to go throughout the week.

Recipes to fill you up.

When your hungry, maybe you just really want a drink.

Subway with all salads please—avoiding fattening processed meats—your going to feel it in your belly straight away.

I had a great day and I did not think of food at all" you exclaimed.

Well you ate, but that you were not preoccupied by having large amounts. You were busy in between things and so it ought to be like that.

Food is one of the greatest pleasures of life, but there are others and so we can get the best parts in moderation while still being able to appreciate food without overindulging and losing that appreciation for food, but taking for granted by the intake of large doses.

Genetic metabolism myth

The ancient Christian fast for example—Wednesday and Friday. No cheese and meat.

Regular fast is important, this is in synchronisation with the little fasts everyday routine I recommended where, you should never become addicted to certain foods, but find the discipline to regularly abstain especially from complex compounded food like the meats and [processed cheeses.

Just by temporarily eliminating these foods on a regular bases could mean the difference whether you are always healthy and always sick.

Great recipes Primary ingredients.

Basil, spring onion, shallots, garlic, balsamic vinegar and olive oil.

All these primary ingredients have anti infection properties or disinfectant properties by constantly cleaning your body.

Why people have great metabolisms and don't get fat, can be found in the fact that they burn it with the use of lemon grass, gingers and other hot spices that clean the blood of toxins and therefore reduce weight.

You cannot think of losing weight without having to look at your total holistic health.

There is simply no short cut, in the world of fads and convenience that do not want to criticise your unhealthy eating habits and in a day and age of msg and chemically processed food that contribute to those thunder thighs and cellulite, we need to be self empowered and nurture our intuition and intellect to take control of our lifestyle and health as much as we can and if we fall, find the template to compensate, through a system of compensations ensuring that there is a certain amount of consistency into your balanced lifestyle regime and then always sort to incrementally improve them, by making for example doing effortless stretches and exercises in the morning while preserving your energy for the day and even gaining energy to your day. Doing a 5 minute knee to chest before a shower is a great habit to have that will built resistance and resilience to your busy and stressful day and will also synthesise your propensity to metabolise more effectively. This is also the most effective and economical and practical way to lasting weight loss

Do away with the frozen fish and frozen chips and fast food chips when you can fry chips at home with olive oil that is not fattening. Olive oil provides the anti aging properties associated better complexions. Now do you want to have extra virgin olive oil in your cupboard and use it also for oil. It is a myth that this oil is too thick for cooking.

This is lubricant for your cells to grow and reproduce healthily.

It should not even be called the essential fats our bodies need for good maintenance , it is only something they see and identify wrongly as being so. Marketers once propagated a fat free diet is good for your health as the only criteria to achieving weight loss without distinguishing between the good fats that are actually needed so that you do not become fat.

Traditionally,Mediterranean woman who fill their belly's with the stuff remain beautifully healthy and thin, are a testimony to the fact. Olives olives olives , tomatoes tomatoes. Accustomize your taste buds to these foods and this will do wonders. If you do not have a taste for them you have a distorted and sick taste bud that needs to be cured and reassessed-- no kidding. If you do not ground and soil your culinary appreciation of essential staple foods that are virtually applied to all your dishes, then forget about losing weight or enjoying a robust healthy weight loss lifestyle.

Octopus with vinegar and lemon and olive oil, you can see that these items self clean the food before we even digest it and can even make your vegetables more appealing. Try a carrot dipped with lemon and eat in interchangeably with an olive-- taste good? U bet. These foods are made for you to eat in combinations. For example gourmet food is impossible without the shallots and garlics etc

The closest parallel to this in our world is the hotdog with onions.

The onions do allot to clean the meat, but in this case not enough as some sausages are too processed, but they add taste. If you feel like a hot dog no reason not too every so often as your lifestyle allows it

Mediterranean snack lunch.

Fetta cheese , tomatoes, cucumbers, kalamata olives or spanish olives, wood oven 98% fat free bread , and maybe some celery and carrot.

Spread olive oil and maybe some salt and pepper and eat the tomatoes with basil

The bread will fill you up so that you do not get hungry within the 3 hours after eating until dinner.

But it is important to eat well and to a certain extent, to your hearts content.

Obvious better alternative to bake beans and prepared noodles, which whenever I have a certain popular brand, puffs me up and gives me a headache because the woman of the house sometimes try to economise by buying absolute junk.

Spend money on food especially prawns and salmon which do not go through the same hormone antibiotic process as the meats go through. Buy plenty of mustard and chilli, they clean everything and most importantly add taste to make them more digestible.

One of the best economically and cost effective fast foods to buy is the veg subway.

This is a medicinal guilt free and tasty treat all in one.

No meat but with all salads and this means all salads, capsicum, onions, carrots, pickles and chilis but make sure you put on your favourite sauces for flavour and the unhealthy cheese helps but the chilli kills all its negative effects. You not purging the food content but neutralising its bacterial and acidic quality that impedes the metabolic process.

This dish Still comprises a fantastic balanced meal whenever your feeling guilty and want something that is good for your health while enjoying the taste of the roll.

note

It is important that you buy home Australian garlic as it does not go through all the bleaching, gassing and radiation as do the imports. Or garlic made from your local region no matter where you live.

Learning to identify freshness is paramount in this day and age of agri business.

The rosemary sandwich

Buy canned Italian tuna with rosemary flavour—which is the white tuna, better quality than the rest.

Cut Australian organic garlic, there are no exceptions and put also shallots and tomato.

Your thinking this is just a quick off shoot way to make a sandwich healthy without tasting good, but the reality is the shallots and the garlic complement the food and make it gourmet tasting, this is the secret of food.

Gone are the day with the battered schnitzel and boring vegetables with no sauces on them, there is no more reason why people did not eat their vegetables any more. They present the integral ingredient to make food tasty when combined with the right ingredients. In this day and age time is rare, however when you add the factor of health, I hour preparing food has lasting benefits. If you made enough you can have it for lunch the next day by having it cold.

For example rice dishes, start simmering onions and shallots and then add tomatoes and and salmon. This is a very economical dish that is called a risotto and to make the salmon taste exquisite put in asparagus. Asparagus on its own is crap, but now you have placed and positioned the right foods within the right dishes. You as the new found chef will possess a pronounced ability to adapt and be creative in what you can put into your risotto and rice is very cheap and it is very quick to make.

Now I am going to go into practical greek recipes that combine vegetables, meats and seafood is very healthy ways, that still satisfy the hunger and fill your belly, but with what you body needs to function and thrive.

Dieting is not limiting food intake but selecting types of foods to properly intake.

It is not a fad or a trick to lose weight forever, but diet is indistinguishably linked to lifestyle and a healthy view to life mentally physically and spiritually

Eating less only suppresses your appetite and is inherently unhealthy.

This the basis of this little ebook.

You will not get a comprehensive list of recipes, but the recipes I do mention, are the most easiest to integrate into the diet and lifestyle.

If you have already eaten about enough, have some teas or some fruit or nuts. But make a limitation on snacks with your compensatory conditions so to average out the positive of your lifestyle routine.

This is important, that apart from the fact that you ought to eat well when you do eat, there is the obvious case when you eat out of stress or succumb to depression dictated eating, where we compensate for our life imbalance and when we are not really hungry and still excessively eat.

When you are preoccupied too often with eating snacks always between meals, you know that you need to find a hobby and get busy walking around, and refraining from eating cakes and banana bread with your coffee. However you can reward yourself from time to time when you know so far in the week you have eaten the correct foods, for example, bean salad or lentil soup etc.

prepare some pasta and some salad and have them in the fridge and then when it is time to have a salad, open a can of quality tuna and then add in all the ingredients, mix in a little pasta with the salad and put in all the fat burners in the salad. Buy fresh beans and throw them in the mix, remember with all these ingredients, this is a delicious dish.

Focusing of cleaning your body is maintaining your body, like some gelato after a heavy meal helps digestion, it is ok to have some icecream but do not over do it. Have fruit with it though and the icecream will taste better.

Even though gellato is best for digestion and neutralising the fat producing acids of the dish, ice cream can form a similar function if eaten in low proportion and with salad and especially with homemade ice cream.

When your hungry at night, have some chips, and every now and then maybe 2 nights a week have medicinal tea like chamomile and this will prevent you from seeing the doctor by maintaining your most valuable asset and will clean your tummy at night so there is no dreaded bloating. An essay and thesis can be written how herbal tea at night will set your metabolism with blazing guns running for the next day. It is literally detoxifying your stomach with such a powerful force that is it literally cleaning out your stomach from those dreaded fat producing acids in your gut.

Remembering the focus is not repression which is unrealistic and that will back fire latter but moderation and dissipation from time to time or giving in, knowing that all in all you are averaging the week out.

It was never a problem to have a few bad snacks here and there, the issue always has been the attitude to eating and tendencies to eating certain types of foods. This is a major obstacle that needs to be faced. We are looking for effortless consistency through incremental improvement gradually until you have sustained positive habit forming behaviours across the whole board and throughout the course of the week.

Why meat when beans.

It is funny that tacos taste just as good or not even better with beans as they meant to be.

In this over eating society we are obsessed with meat, it is important to complement this with beans and a spinach dish I will divulge to you in a moment.

Spinach with broad beans

Packed with olive oil and salt and some vinegar, your going to be shocked when you eat this with onion and bread to fill up this goodness, it will be addictive and tasty and you are going out of your way in improving your physical and mental states and of course your waste.

More energy, better moods, no worries about your belly and olive virgin oil for your skin.

It is like all those products that make promises that it will improve your looks when it is also very important to look good by eating what is right for your inside.

For a little more add tuna with olive oil in it.

It is the only way I find to eat that valuable spinach like poppy I believed that spinach gave you incredible energy and it does. This form of energy is the same fat burning energy you are looking for, if I may for a moment simplify the process.

It is agreed that preparing beans with boiled spinach topped with extra virgin olive oil after it has been cooked with lemon and salt is a dish that everyone will like. This is the medicine, the facial toner, the daily food preventative and mood stabiliser for the brain all in one and your paying virtually little money. And maximised good taste. But to fill to suit you must have it with bread. This is a Greek Mediterranean dish.

Are u disciplined to have that veg juice every now and then?

It is a sacrifice to go away from your pre-packaged smoothies and have a veg juice, but sometimes we need to as a little detox from all the crap we eat everyday.

Our body contains inherent signals when we over eat which leads to in some woman the unhealthy and damaging response to regurgitate it back up.

When we eat something that does not agree with our stomach, we should listen to our bodies because it is by this way it forces us to clean our bodies and stay in tune with what our bodies require of us. Only through this way we learn and retain the nutrition. This whole book has demonstrated that simply eating fruit after dinner would neutralise any fatty feeling you perceived after the meal. Remember your senses can be tainted whereby you had a normal meal and feel it to be too fat. You must get some help and support and reassurance that you are not. If you genuinely feel you had a bad meal and reacted badly to it, then on top of the fruit have herbal tea. That'll kill it.

When we have those pre packaged prepared noodles with all those msgs , your going to feel bloated, your temperature will go up a little and all this so that body's immune system can slowly filter out all the toxins that has been ingested into your body.

To gain this new lifestyle is imperative that you self observe in this fashion what your body is going through after a meal and how to counter it.

It is up to you to assist the immune system in its fight against the ailment and bad food it is fighting to clean up by eating fruit and eating gelato and having some herbal tea, to calm the stomach and help it digest the bad elements of the food, this will also heal any fever or slight sick feeling you gained from the bad food.

That is why I am an advocate of always drinking water when your binging out. So that you clean everything you put in your body. Just now I had two coffees and the coffee maker put too much milk and my belly is upset and I feel a little agitated. I am now cancelling its effects by having plenty of water and when I am out of this cafe, I will buy an apple. Seeing how I go I might even have some herbal tea at night.

So if you feel bad afterwards and you have been known to be a bulimic.

Understand that by regurgitating it back up, you lost the opportunity to learn from your mistake and by learning to compensate and self clean your actions with the use of food and exercise. This lifestyle this book presents will gain you a high threshold and consistency of health promoting behaviours and perspectives that will prevent you from falling into the those treacherous fluctuations that are characteristic of diet fads and those extreme compensations you may respond to after a series or single incident bad binge experience that never address the problem nor streamline your diet lifestyle through at least a series of chastised compensation checks where at least after a bad dish choice you would compensate it with a piece of fruit and water so to ease metabolism of excess and aid digestion. You are then in control and see the bigger picture, you have perfectly rationalised that gut wrenching feelings after eating as probably a bad food eating experience and you have learnt that you can cancel its effects through a series of little detoxes that are without effort. Now who is really in control?

When you go through the ordeal and the guilt of eating something disagreeable, do not get overly consumed with this idea. Rather focus on cleaning your body with plenty filtered water, fruit or gelato and maybe a few stretches with the mental conviction and determination of trying to improve you bouts of appetites next time round.

Don't worry your metabolism will deal with it , as long as you are averaging off and consistently making some changes within your eating regime, mistakes here and there find a way to compliment and improve our routine or they simply maintain them by making us more resolved and stronger about the choices of food we make and places we choose to go to eat.

Remember it is not your genes but your environment and lifestyle that needs to be amended. Otherwise thinking your born a certain way is a form of negative reinforcement that never addresses the real issue. We are born with different types of bodies, but no body is born to be fat. The latest genetic research always affirms this fact even though sometimes genes downplays the role of environment because of the entrenched conflicts of interests and the vested interests in patented medicine and gene mapping. Don't be fooled.

Mediterranean Food Guide Pyramid.

Remember cooking recipes are the perfect sythesis to ensuring you are eating all the important foods necessary to begin your new outlook and lifestyle.
Start keeping a diary of what you eat.

A little food appreciation goes along way to completely shift your world-view and attitude to foods as a precious life sustaining sustenance, medicine, cosmetic complimenter, as a natural replenisher that no expensive cream can ever replace or compare.
HERE is a little dose--

The traditional diets of the Mediterranean region were mainly based on a diverse menu of plant sources, including fruits, vegetables, whole grains, beans, nuts and seeds. In North Africa, couscous, vegetables and legumes form the center of the diet; in Southern Europe it was rice, polenta, pasta, potatoes with vegetables and legumes.

In the Eastern Mediterranean, bulgur and rice together with vegetables and legumes, such as chick peas, constitute the core of many meals. Throughout the Mediterranean bread is a staple in the diet and is eaten without butter or margarine.

The Mediterranean diet delivers as much as 40% of total daily calories from fat, yet the associated incidence of cardiovascular diseases is significantly decreased because the fat comes mainly from olive oil and fish.

As a monosaturated fatty acid, olive oil does not have the same cholesterol-raising effect of saturated fats. Olive oil is also a good source of antioxidants.

Eating fish a few times per week benefits the Mediterranean people by increasing the amount of "omega-3 fatty acids", something that the rest of the developed societies don't get enough of.
note

Also a consideration here is that when chickens are left to graze and feed on the natural environment without intervention of hormones, chemicals, pellets and other manufactured feed for livestock, then it has been shown that in Crete the chickens there have high levels of omega three, because of the natural non commoditizing reality of open livestock feed in the Mediterranean regions.

This merely stresses importance of saving more money when eating out to opt for the free range chicken is more nutritional.

your body is always trying to flush out all the chemicals, synthetic compounds and complex fats associated predominately with processed and prepared foods. If you body is more consumed with cleaning rather than processing nutrition, your metabolism is decreased and your propensity to keep thin is compromised. But remember never from a single event, this is why you see those eating allot and never loss weight is because they do have regular bouts of fasting and eating moderately and because they listen to their body, they are acutely aware of the best time to start eating to hearts content.

The reason for this is that this experience of eating allot compliments their moderate eating and active lifestyle, you cannot lose weight or keep thin unless you are well nourished. Sudden deprivation of eating by people overweight will not work for anybody. Those people that lose weight via cold turkey, will find it harder to keep the weight loss as they may not be mentally prepared for a lifestyle that is suited to their new weight so to sustain it.

Those that have these show off bouts of eating plenty know their limits and are in control of their weight through these inbuilt control mechanisms of little fasts, little detoxs, little times when you do not eat in the morning, times when you should drink rather than eat, and most importantly they are not addicted to bad food or those that made a note of where the coffee made them bloat or sick and actually investigate and get angry how to take control and resolve it.Oh it was the processed milk, ok next time I will order a long black and poor in the milk myself solved. Better still black tea and avoid coffee makers mixing in too much milk with its highly complex compound mix of chemicals and crap that is in it. A self reflectory state is paramount. You are self observing, but remember, it is a comfortable experience once you get rid of some bad habits-- like having a piece of dessert everyday without varying your food.

Without knowledge, we cannot build up the anger to realise and resolve what in fact made us sick when we ate out. we instead attribute to an allergy and a random reaction or disposition and therefore we do not have the impetus and motivation to make the correction or the adjustment in our behaviour.

This is essential in your lifestyle that you understand the causes of your imbalances rather than attributing to non existent. It is only through this procedure that we can make the proper recourse and adjustments throughout the day and course of our lifestyle routine. This also encompasses what it means to be human, to react, to respond to adjust, to constantly strive to reaching homeostasis or equilibrium in our body. If it is making you sick or fat, god gave us brain to discern it is not natural and so just get out from the fire. Do not be afraid to let the resturant or cafe know how you feel too.

More on food culture___

Even though it is hard to get natural chicken products, they are attainable, and the rest, the immune system will handle when we ensure that you do ingest regular fruit and vegetables, ensuring they are made in Australia or from your local country and fresh and even though they may contain traces of chemicals, that is why god invented the liver cause he foresaw the destruction man has reaped on the natural environment and our primary reliance on unnutritional deficient processed food because todays society encourages us and indoctrinates us with quickly prepared food and instant gratification and instant cures . A healthy lifestyle always requires effort, but the pain of slow incremental forming behaviours is relative small and through your own gradual efforts and with time you will reach a state of comfort as you will witness how better you'll feel. You will find a way as long as you persist and never give up and when you do fall out at times, make it a life changing experience to help you reshape your attitude and outlook to pave a continually better lifestyle that is more healthier each time.

But do not obsess in always having chemical free chicken, for example,just be wary and conscious of the choices you can make. Sometimes it is not always feasible economically to buy organic produce. Although I will always stress on having eggs as free range and at the very least the chickens used were not subjugated to courses of pellet feed. Free range eggs have a better omega 3 content and so they are worth the extra expense. However you can get away with non organic vegetables, as long as they are in season. Organic grapes may be worth it, especially when you can first hand the powder pesticide residue in non organic grapes.

N-3 fatty acids may have <u>health benefits</u> and are considered <u>essential fatty acids</u>, meaning that they cannot be synthesized by the human body but are vital for normal <u>metabolism.</u>

Eating red meat sparingly also seems to increase health. There is a general consensus among health professionals that the **Mediterranean diet** is healthier than the North European and American diets because of the higher consumption of grains such as spaghetti, fruits, vegetables, legumes, nuts, and olive oil.

The main issue here is that the western world is addicted to meat products and especially processed products.

Unfortunately in this day in age of agribusiness, food is passed as if a commodity and therefore the treatment as such demeans the quality of food in its production, distribution and finally its delivery,demonstration and presentation.

Understanding the nature of food and finance, of franchises should incite us to really reflect on the quality of the food we ingest.

Mediterranean diets and all local sustaining regional farming communities were rich with nutrients because local communities lived in harmony with the natural surroundings, the local markets, which produced fresh produce and produced a natural society where all participated in the food culinary process. Sorting preparing arranging, cooking and delivering. Disease and obesity were low because the Mediterranean diet provided the sufficiency that replenished the deficiency and excess that is associated and characterised with the cause of these diseases in the first place.

So the Mediterranean diet is not simply another diet, but an example of a diet that is indistinguishable to balance and lifestyle as small farming techniques always most certainly makes more nutritional food and freshly available food is imperative when today apples could be stocked in freezes for a year and are full of pesticides and compromise our health.

Today we need to acquire more effort to gain food because of all the processed food that has evaded our whole lives, however it emphasises one important feature, the ability to collect fresh food, to prepare it and to cook it. This is not a diet routine or sequence but a very attitude of our outlook to life that is not fad diet but a ways to ones every day existence.

So the Mediterranean diet is also an example of a diet or rather a lifestyle and outlook.

The main feature of the Mediterranean diet is not the food but the philosophy that food produced in season and food enjoyed with family in the outdoors sustains the necessary balance necessary to avoid being sick and avoid being unhealthy.

Today, in the western world, only a few food companies control all production of food and therefore have made fresh good food inaccessible or made cheaper if we purchased fast food rather than government subsidising good healthy farmed food.

So now food is destroyed in order to keep prices high and to protect import markets for in superior products that put virtue of transportation and blatant economics ahead of people and their health.

We are bombarded to the exposure of chemicals and other impurities in even our fruits and vegetables, remember the treated ones still have some nutrition, however the organic ones are better. But if you do not have the money always to buy organic , don't worry because mainstream vegetables are good as long as they are fresh and you find a good local retailer. You will know from the smell and the look of a fruit if whether a fruit or vegetable is in season and therefore have very little chemicals used in them. Most importantly have faith god made them strong enough to overwhelm any impurities that may be in them. Photo aura imaging has shown that even in inorganic fruits and vegetables, the aura and energy vibration frequency within them still shows they are living breathing organisms filled with nutrients and minerals good for our health.

Remember to avoid imported fruits and vegetables because they are irradiated with radiation and sometimes gassed like garlic is, so they can make it into your country.

One wonders if man has successfully made garlic in the minus in terms of nutritional value, by bleaching, by gassing and irritating products before they come into the country. I would avoid these anyway and seek organic garlic. Or if not locally produced garlic. Buy american if you live in america for example.

So when farms are dedicated to fast food chains for its production, good food available at affordable costs are marginalised over the burgeoning agribusiness of exploitation .

This should infuriate within us all the motivation, to do better, to make sure food is our lifestyle rather than the other way around.

Another issue is that food cuisine is not part of everyday culture, it is commoditized as a form of diet program on some chef show, instead of the recipe being an integral part of your lifestyle and your daily culture.

It so happens that these eating habits result in low levels of heart and other chronic diseases. Some of its key characteristics include:

- In traditional Mediterranean diets, **fruits and vegetables** are locally grown and often consumed raw or minimally processed. This may be a crucial factor given our present understanding of the potential protective factors of dietary fiber, antioxidants, and other micronutrients found in plant foods.

- Olive oil, high in monounsaturated fat, is a good source of antioxidants and is the area's principle source of fat. Evidence suggests that Mediterranean diets are about 40% fat, when bodies like the American Heart Association recommend 30%. However, it is very low in saturated and polyunsaturated fat. A high intake of fat in the form of olive oil in the traditional Greek diet does not have any apparent negative health consequences. It is believed that olive oil is neutral with respect to effects of serum cholesterol. However, current research has found olive oil and its high monounsaturated fat may actually increase HDL (good) cholesterol, but has little effect on LDL (bad) cholesterol.

- **Dairy products** from a variety of animals like goats, sheep, buffaloes, cows, and camels, primarily in the form of cheese and yogurt, are traditionally consumed in low to moderate amounts. In the entire region, fresh milk is consumed sparingly and meals are usually accompanied by wine or water. Research suggests that the live bacterial cultures of yogurt may have contributed to the region's good health.

- Meat and especially **red meat** is avoided. Fish consumption varies between countries but overall is slightly higher than red meat. There is evidence to suggest that red meat is associated with colon cancer, prostate cancer, and heart disease, possibly due to carcinogens formed from cooking. Furthermore, animal products contain no fiber or antioxidants and may displace plant based foods that do contain these important elements.

- Throughout the Mediterranean **wine** is drunk in moderation and usually taken with meals. For men moderation is two glasses per day, for women moderation is one glass per day. That is important because current research suggests there is a correlation between alcohol intake and a reduction in heart disease. The Mediterranean diet food pyramid is not based solely on either the weight or the percentage of calories intake. It is rather a combination of these that is meant to convey relative proportions and a general sense of frequency of servings, as well as an indication of which foods to favor in a healthy Mediterranean-style diet.

So, when you come to Greece, partake of the local eating habits and try to adopt some or all them when you return home. This may turn out to be a much more important long-term legacy of your stay here than the memories, the experiences, and the photos.

Spanish diet shows how people keep thin"

Spanish researchers have concluded that people who follow the Mediterranean diet are less likely to gain weight as they grow older.

Researchers from the University of Las Palmas de Gran Canaria and University of Navarra in Spain studied over 10,000 Spanish men and women with an average age of 38 years at the start of the study.

Subjects had their diets analyses and were each given a "Mediterranean dietary score" which indicated how closely their diet is to a pure Mediterranean diet.

"Adherence to the Mediterranean dietary pattern is significantly associated with reduced weight gain. This dietary pattern can be recommended to slow down age-related weight gain."

a little history of Mediterranean cuisine

The Mediterranean countries knew of the existence and use of butter, but they didn't use it that much, probably for two reasons, a) they used olive oil and b) it may have been impractical given their lifestyle and weather. However, there were mixed opinions on butter – the Greek poet *Anaxandrides* called the *Thracians " boutyrophagoi"* (butter eaters) and he wasn't being nice about it, but *Pliny* the Roman, on the other hand, felt that it was a most elegant food eaten by barbarous nations.

During the Renaissance, the Scandinavian countries became the most significant butter exporters and thanks, probably, to their cooler climates but also to superior feeding, extraordinarily good vegetation and good old-fashioned animal husbandry it thrived. They started exporting significantly around the 12th century. After Rome's demise butter was commonly used throughout Europe even though not considered a luxury item then. As with all good things, the peasants ate it first and it took some time before the upper classes realised what they were missing. The Brits, in particular, took to eating butter very enthusiastically.

The overuse of butter is a major contributor to obesity and heart problems. The primary ingredient to use in cooking is olive oil and butter only proportionately with certain dishes.

Butter has its place. Unfortunately the market driven food market has made it too abundant.

Garlic Cures

Garlic's Special Properties

Fresh garlic has many active constituents including alliin, allicin, alliinase and unique sulfur compounds. Allicin and the sulfur compounds of garlic are the ingredients primarily responsible for garlic's potency as an antibiotic, anti-viral and a fungicide and for its use in treating high blood pressure, lowering cholesterol, and for helping to prevent certain types of cancer, as well as its use as an immune stimulant. Allicin is a strong antibiotic agent produced when the alliin and alliinase are merged together, as happens when a fresh garlic clove is crushed or chewed.

GARLIC TEA FOR COUGHS
Marco, a well known soux chef in Santa Monica, California, gave us this simple soup recipe for nagging coughs. This is an old Mexican recipe from Marco's mother that aided him and his siblings' flu/cold recovery process.

Recipe:
Cut a garlic cube into quarters and add to two 2 quarts of H2O.
Boil on low flame for at least one hour.
Strain and sip slowly.

Believe or not, this warm garlic soup has a very pleasant taste!

HISTORY OF GARLIC
Garlic has a long history in folklore as a protector from disease and. Hippocrates, the father of modern medicine, used garlic in infectious diseases and particularly prescribed it for intestinal disorders.

12th century German mystic Hildegarde von Bingen recommended simmering garlic in water for twenty minutes and drinking the "tea" for bronchial problems like asthma. This treatment is still in use in many cultures. Three cloves of garlic in boiling water is also recommended as a topical cure for athlete's foot. Additionally, garlic was used extensively in the battlefields during World War I (1914-1918) to treat and dress wounds and infections. Being a natural antibiotic and widely available, it was the most effective antiseptic available at the time.

HEALING POWERS OF GARLIC:

Garlic has been used in herbal medicine to treat asthma, deafness, leprosy, bronchial, congestion, hardening of arteries, fevers, worms and liver and gall bladder trouble. Herbal books list it being useful in Leucoderma, leprosy, piles, worms, catarrhal disorders and cough. Additionally, it is reported that garlic is good for the heart, stimulates appetite, and is an energy tonic.

Garlic's unpleasant odor is due to its sulphur content. This mineral is contained to a greater degree in its volatile oil, which has remarkable medicinal virtues.

Juice of garlic has a most beneficial effect on the entire system as it helps dissolve an accumulation of mucus in the sinus cavities, bronchial tubes and the lungs. It also helps expel poison from body through pores of the skin.

SUMMARY
* Garlic is a gastric stimulant & helps with digestion.
* It acts as an anti flatulent, carminative and diaphoretic.
* It stimulates the kidneys and is diuretic in nature.
* It is a tonic, giving strength & vitality
* It is an expectorant having a special effect on the bronchial and pulmonary secretions.
* It is beneficial for eyes & brain.
* It helps to heal fractured bones (also see comfrey poultices)
* It is a great antiseptic.
* It has allicin, which has the property to destroy germs which are not killed by penicillin. As such, it is a very powerful germicidal.
* It rehabilitates sexual malfunctions.
* It improves functional activity of heavy smokers.
* Half a raw garlic clove a day can increase body activity to dissolve blood clots, thereby preventing heart attacks and strokes.
* A couple of raw garlic cloves daily can bring blood cholesterol levels down in heart patients.

Mediterranean lifestyle book has provided one example how the medicinal effects of food, for example garlic in this instance, are the very identical effects needed to keep the body in a condition necessary to have a healthy weight. Learning about food and how food can prevent disease provides us with the knowledge and weaponry needed to compensate for the crap that many times we cannot help digesting in our body.

For example, garlic destroying clots can clear the way for blood to circulate properly and this means an enhanced metabolic rate necessary to achieve a low weight level. The body is interconnected.

Apple cider vinegar

Apple Cider Vinegar, that wonderful old-timers home remedy, cures more ailments than any other folk remedy -- we're convinced! From the extensive feedback we've received over the past 8 years, the reported cures from drinking Apple Cider Vinegar are numerous. They include cures for allergies, sinus infections, acne, high cholesterol, flu, chronic fatigue, candida, acid reflux, sore throats, contact dermatitis, arthritis, and gout. Apple Cider Vinegar also breaks down fat and is widely used to lose weight. It has also been reported that a daily dose of apple cider vinegar in water has high blood pressure under control in two weeks!

. Mead is a unique and rare beverage made by fermenting honey, it's the oldest fermented drink known to mankind, named Ambrosia Nectar of the Gods by the ancient Greeks. The Vikings believed it to be an aphrodisiac, the groom and wedding guests indulging it for one month, hence the Honeymoon! The McLaren Vale's Maxwell Winery sits comfortably at the forefront of Australian Meads, and this Honey labelled is always refreshing with a surprising length of flavour, even when mixed with dry ginger ale (a favourite long drink locally in McLaren Vale). Chilled with crushed ice in summer it exhibits citrus peel and dried apricot characters, whilst it can also be used creatively in cooking.

The following are greek recipes that can revolve around your new lifestyle.

Primary ingredients you may want to have everyday

Extra virgin olive oil

Balsamic vinegar and apple cider vinegar

Shallots

A basil plant or buying basil

Australian garlic if in australian . or from your local farmer

Onions

olives

natural honey.

Thes ingredients are usually associated with a platter of food eaten interchangeably. Very nice with bread and will fill your appetite. The fat killing effects of this platter is amazing and learning to enjoy it with tomatoes and cucumbers with a little feta or haloumi cheese, make this irristible.

Use 98% fat free bread, wood oven bread should be added in meals that are no always too feeling and eating them with onions or shallots.

Notice all these ingredients mention self clean and neutral any negative effects of any food, eg.
Sometimes seafood has mercury and so olive oil and onions will help kidneys neutralise this effect.

Medicine diet and lifestyle go hand in hand. Enjoy Enjoy Enjoy!!

Now for the recipes! The backbone of your lifestyle.

GREEK CHICKEN RECIPE

Ingredients (serves 4)

- 750g chat or kipfler potatoes, skin on, cut into medium pieces
- 8 small chicken thighs on the bone, skin on
- 2 tsp sweet paprika
- 2 Spanish onions, quartered
- 1 red capsicum, cut into strips
- 1 yellow capsicum, cut into strips
- 3 garlic cloves, crushed
- 40ml (2 tbs) olive oil
- 1 tbs chopped fresh oregano
- 400g can diced tomatoes
- 12 black olives
- Chopped flat-leaf parsley, to serve
- 1 cup crumbled fetta, to serve

Method

1. Preheat oven to 200°C.
2. Cook potatoes in a large pan of boiling water for 5 minutes. Drain and set aside to cool.
3. Pat dry the chicken, place in a large baking dish and toss in the paprika.
4. Add the onion, capsicum, garlic and potatoes. Drizzle with oil, sprinkle with oregano and season well. Bake for 30 minutes. Add tomatoes and olives, basting chicken with the juices, and cook for 15 minutes.
5. Serve with parsley and fetta.

Greek White Bean Salad

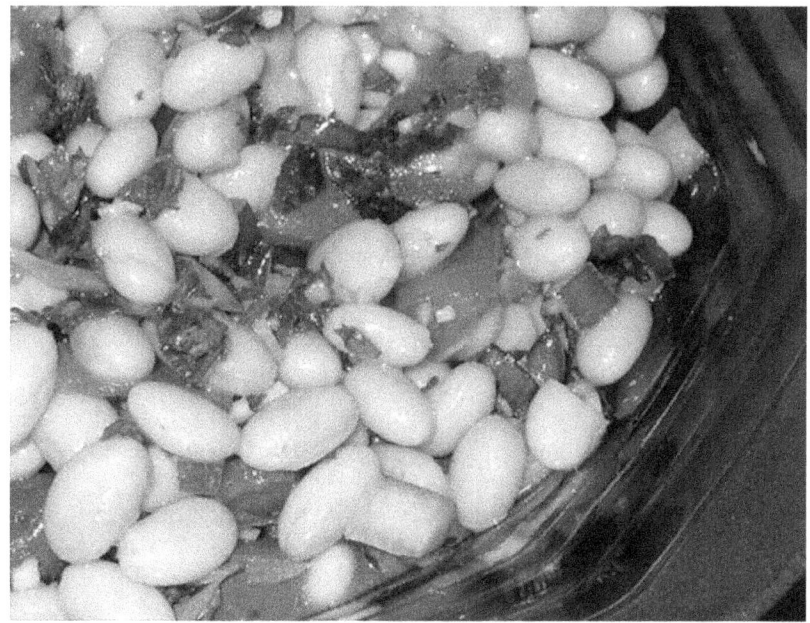

4 (15 ounce) cans white beans , drained
1 (15 ounce) can stewed tomatoes , drained
1/2 cup fresh basil
1/2 cup fresh mint
1/2 cup fresh parsley
4 garlic cloves , pressed
1 red onion , chopped
1 teaspoon lemon juice (to taste)
1/3 cup olive oil , to taste
salt and pepper
Directions:

1
Mix all ingredients, chill 1 hour.
2
Enjoy. Simple and enjoyable I guarantee.

YEMISTA STUFFED VEGETABLES RECIPE

Ingredients:

- 2 large green bell peppers
- 5 medium zucchini + 1 small zucchini
- 3 medium eggplant
- 1 large potato
- 5 large ripe tomatoes
- 1 medium onion, grated
- 3/4 cup of fresh parsley, finely chopped
- 2 cups + 1 tablespoon of long-grain rice
- 1 teaspoon of salt
- 1/2 teaspoon of pepper
- 1 cup of olive oil
- 3 tablespoons of water

Preparation:

Wash all vegetables well, and peel the potato.

Trim & Scoop Out Vegetables:

Use a large bowl to hold the vegetable pulp.

- Tomatoes: Cut a cap off the top of tomatoes. Using a teaspoon, scoop out tomato pulp and put in a bowl. Set tomatoes and caps aside.
- Bell peppers: Cut a cap off the top of the peppers, scoop out seeds, and rinse well. Set peppers and caps aside.
- Potato: cut a thick slice off the potato lengthwise. Scoop out interior of potato and put in the bowl with the other vegetables, leaving a 1/8 inch shell. Set potato and top aside.
- Eggplants: cut off the top with stem. Using a spoon, scoop out eggplant pulp and add to bowl with other vegetables. Set eggplants and tops aside.
- Zucchini: trim tops of the 5 large zucchini, and using a spoon handle, scoop out zucchini pulp and add to bowl. Set zucchini and tops aside. Cut the small zucchini into 8 slices and set aside.

Make the Stuffing

Using a vegetable grater (or the large grate on a cheese grater), grate all the pulp that was scooped out from the vegetables, as well as the tops of the zucchini and eggplant, and place in a large bowl.

Wash the rice, and add to the bowl. Add grated onion, parsley, salt, pepper, and all but 2 tablespoons of olive oil. Mix well. The stuffing mix will be soupy.

Stuff the Vegetables

Using a teaspoon, fill the vegetables to within 1/2 inch of the top. The rice will expand when cooked so take care not to overfill. Place caps on top, using the zucchini slices for the eggplant and zucchini.

Cooking

Place the vegetables in a 14 x 11 inch (or equivalent) baking or roasting pan. The tomatoes should be placed upright, and the other vegetables should be placed on their sides. They should fit snugly in the pan.

There will be a little oil left in the bottom of the bowl. Add 3 tablespoons of water and pour the mixture into the pan with the vegetables. Drizzle the vegetables with the remaining olive oil (2 tablespoons).

Place vegetables in a cold oven and heat to 480F (250C). When the liquid starts to boil (about 10-15 minutes), reduce heat to 355F (180C) and cook for one hour.

Allow the vegetables to sit for 20 minutes before serving. Stuffed vegetables are served warm or at room temperature and are excellent the second day.

Yield: serves 4-6

In Greek: σπανακόριζο or σπανακόρυζο, pronounced spah-nah-KOH-ree-zoh

This is the traditional recipe for this delicious dish that is a warming and hearty meal in itself or it can be served as a side dish with a light entree. Try topping with a sprinkle of crumbled feta.

Prep Time: 15 minutes

Cook Time: 35 minutes

Total Time: 50 minutes

SPANAKOPIZO RECIPE.

Another way to use spinach in a dish with rice in a delicious vegetarian meal without meat.

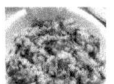

Ingredients:

- 2 1/4 pounds of fresh spinach, chopped, washed, drained
- 1 spring onion, chopped
- 1/3 cups of olive oil
- 1 1/3 cup of water
- 1 1/3 cups of long-grain rice
- 5 1/4 cups of water
- sea salt
- freshly ground pepper
- juice of 1 lemon (about 2 tablespoons)

Preparation:

In a stock pot, sauté the chopped spring onion in the oil over medium heat for 8-10 minutes. Add spinach and 1 1/3 cups of water and cook until the spinach wilts, about 5-7 minutes. Add rice and 5 1/4 cups of water, bring to a boil, and cook for 15 minutes, stirring occasionally. Stir in lemon juice and salt, cook for another 5 minutes and remove from heat. Stir, cover, and let sit for 20 minutes until the dish "melds."

Serve with wedges of lemon and freshly ground pepper.

Prep Time: 20 minutes

Cook Time: 1 hour

FUSSOLAKIA RECIPE

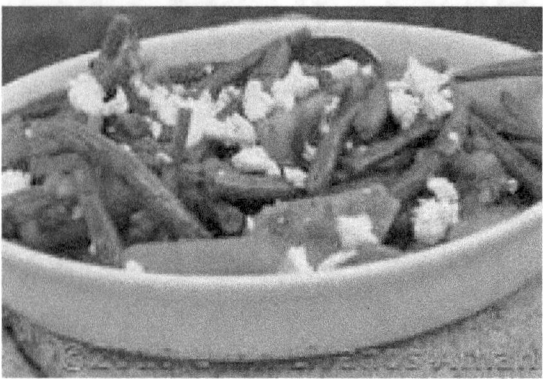

Ingredients:

- 2 lbs. green beans, cleaned and trimmed
- 1/2 cup olive oil
- 1 large onion, diced
- 2 cloves garlic, minced
- 2-3 medium potatoes, cut in large wedges
- A large handful of baby carrots
- 1/2 cup chopped fresh parsley
- 2 tbsp. tomato paste
- 4-5 ripe tomatoes, skinned and crushed (substitute 1 cup canned crushed tomatoes)
- 1½ cups warm water
- 1 tsp. sugar
- 1 tbsp. chopped fresh dill
- Salt and pepper to taste

Preparation:

In a large Dutch oven or pot, heat the olive oil over medium high heat. Add the onion and saute until translucent. Add the garlic and saute until fragrant, about one minute.

Add the green beans, potatoes, and carrots to the pot. Dissolve the tomato paste in the water and add, along with the crushed tomatoes, parsley, and sugar. Lower the heat to medium low and simmer covered for about an hour or until the green beans are tender but not mushy.

In the last ten minutes of cooking, add the chopped fresh dill and season with salt and pepper to taste.

Note: Be sure to monitor your liquid levels while the beans are cooking. You can add a little bit of water if needed.

GREEK PIE SPANAKOPITA RECIPE
looks yummy! Doesn't it.

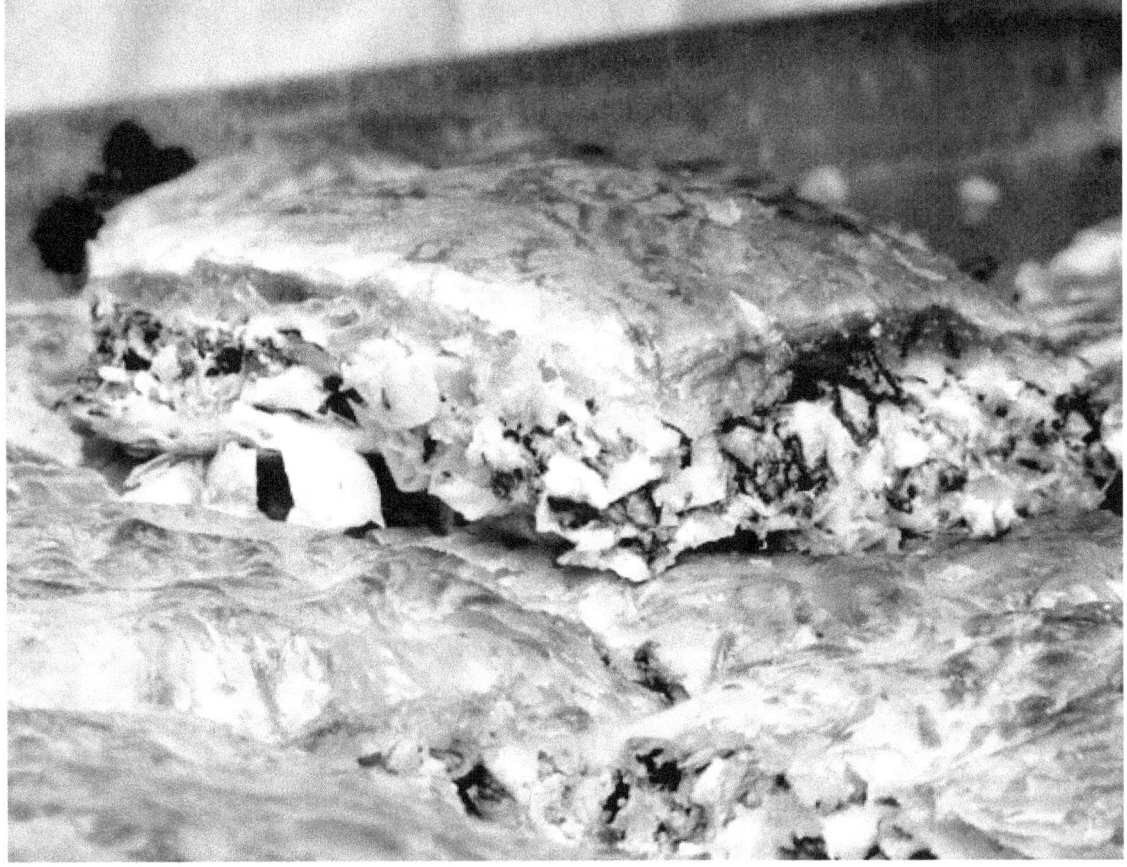

Ingredients:

- 2.5 lbs. spinach, chopped (you can substitute frozen, thawed well)
- 1/2 cup olive oil
- 4 large onions, diced
- 2 bunches green onions, diced (incl. 4 inches green)
- 1/2 cup parsley, chopped
- 1/2 cup fresh dill, chopped (substitute 3 tbsp. dried)
- 1/4 tsp. ground nutmeg
- Salt and freshly ground black pepper to taste
- 1/2 lb. feta cheese, crumbled
- 4 eggs, lightly beaten
- 1/2 lb. ricotta or cottage cheese
- 1/4 cup butter, melted
- 1/4 cup olive oil
- 1 lb. phyllo pastry sheets

Preparation:

Wash and drain the chopped spinach very well. If using frozen spinach, thaw completely and squeeze out excess water. Spinach should be dry.

Heat the olive oil in a deep saute pan or large dutch oven. Saute the onions and green onions until tender. Add the spinach, parsley, and dill and cook for 5 to 10 minutes until the spinach is wilted and heated through. Add the nutmeg and season with salt and pepper.

If using frozen spinach, you will want to cook until excess moisture evaporates. Spinach mixture should be on the dry side.

Remove from heat and set the spinach aside to cool.

In a large mixing bowl, combine the feta, eggs, and ricotta (cottage) cheese. Add the cooled spinach mixture and mix until combined.

Combine the melted butter with the olive oil in a bowl. Using a pastry brush, lightly grease two 9 x 12 rectangular pans.

Unwrap the Phyllo:

Carefully remove the Phyllo roll from the plastic sleeve. Most packages come in 12 x 18 inch sheets when opened fully. Using a scissor or sharp knife, cut the sheets in half to make two stacks of 9x12 inch sheets. To prevent drying, cover one stack with wax paper and a damp paper towel while working with the other.

Prepare the Pita:

Layer about 10 sheets on the bottom of the pan making sure to brush each sheet with the butter/olive oil mixture. Add half of the spinach mixture in an even layer and press with a spatula to flatten.

Layer another 10 sheets on top of the spinach mixture making sure to brush well with butter/olive oil mixture. Repeat the process with the second pan.

Before baking, score the top layer of phyllo (making sure not to puncture filling layer) to enable easier cutting of pieces later. I place the pan in the freezer to harden the top layers and then use a serrated knife.

Bake in a preheated 350 degree oven until the pita turns a deep golden brown. If the pita is frozen when you put it in the oven, you will need approximately 45 minutes cooking time. If fresh, plan for approximately 20 to 25 minutes of cooking time.

BRAZED EGGPLANT WITH POTATO

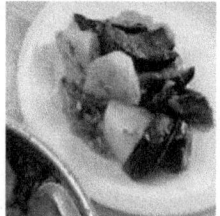

Total Time: 65 minutes

Ingredients:

- 1 pound of eggplant, cut in egg-sized chunks (skin on)
- 2 pounds of potatoes, peeled, cut in chunks
- 3 medium onions, chopped
- 1 bunch of fresh parsley, chopped
- 1 1/2 pounds of fresh tomatoes, pulped (or 2 3/4 cups of pulped stewed tomatoes)
- 1/2 cup of olive oil
- 1 1/4 cups of water + 1/4 cup of water
- 1/2 teaspoon of salt (for sauce)
- 1/2 teaspoon of salt (for vegetables)
- 4 tablespoons of olive oil
- 4 tablespoons of flour

Preparation:

- **To start:** Soak eggplant pieces in water for 30 minutes.

- **Make the sauce:** In a stew pot, combine tomatoes, parsley, onion, 1/2 cup of olive oil, 1

- 1/4 cups of water, and 1/2 teaspoon of salt. Bring to a boil, cover, and cook over medium-high heat for
of water, cover, and cook until the potatoes are done, about 20 minutes.

- **Fry the eggplant:** While the sauce is cooking, drain the eggplant and season with 1/2 teaspoon of salt.
pan over high heat. Dredge the pieces of eggplant in flour and fry until golden brown on all sides. Place fried pie
off.

- Add eggplant to the potatoes and sauce, cover and continue to cook for 10 minutes. Turn off heat and le
serve or store.

- Serve hot, warm, or at room temperature.

- Yield: serves 4

This is a delicious meatless oven casserole that combines the classic tastes of spinach with green
onion, leeks, dill, and feta cheese, combined with giant beans (yigandes) or lima beans. It can also
be made with frozen spinach and, when fresh tomatoes may not be available, canned can be
substituted.

Cook Time: 1 hour, 30 minutes

Total Time: 1 hour, 30 minutes

SPANAKI spinach bean and feta recipe

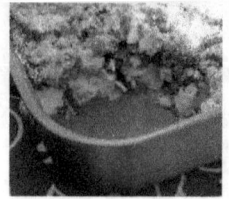

Ingredients:

- 2 1/4 pounds of fresh spinach (or 1 1/2 pounds of frozen chopped spinach)
- 1 pound of yigandes beans (or large lima beans)
- 1 leek, just the white stalk, finely chopped
- 1 bunch of green onions, finely chopped
- 1 bunch of fresh dill, thick stems removed, finely chopped
- 1/2 pound of feta cheese, crumbled
- 3 medium-large ripe tomatoes, peeled and seeded, finely chopped (or a 14.5 oz can of chopped tomatoes, drained)
- 1/2 cup of olive oil
- 3/4 cup of dried bread crumbs
- 2 teaspoons of sea salt
- 1/4 teaspoon of freshly ground pepper

Preparation:

Step 1: Soak the beans in a large bowl of water overnight. The next day, drain and transfer to a large soup pot. Cover with cold water (at least 3 times as much water as beans) and bring to a boil over high heat. When a full boil is reached, reduce heat and cook at a slow boil for 1 hour. Transfer to a colander to drain and set aside.

If using frozen spinach, defrost and skip step 2.

Step 2: Clean spinach well, trim roots, and discard any damaged leaves. Chop coarsely and put in a large bowl or plastic tub.

Step 3: Taking one handful of spinach at a time, squeeze gently but firmly over the sink to remove most excess liquid, and place spinach in a colander. When all the spinach has been squeezed, toss with salt and set aside to drain.

Step 4: Prepare remaining ingredients.

Step 5: Preheat oven to 340°F (170°C). Oil an 11X14 inch (or equivalent) roasting or baking pan (with 2 1/2 inch sides).

Step 6: In a large bowl or plastic tub, combine spinach, onions, leeks, dill, and 1/2 the feta cheese. Toss with hands to mix evenly.

Step 7: Distribute 1/2 the spinach mixture evenly over the bottom of the pan. Add the beans to make an even layer, and place the remaining spinach mixture on top. Sprinkle with remaining cheese, then the chopped tomatoes. Sprinkle with pepper. Pour oil over the top, and finish with an even dusting of bread crumbs.

Step 8: Bake at 340°F (170°C) for about 1 hour 30 minutes. Time will vary depending on the amount of liquid released by the spinach, so check early and keep checking until the bottom of the pan has just a little oil left.

Remove from oven and let sit for 20-30 minutes before serving. This dish is generally served warm or at room temperature.

Yield: serves 6-8, depending on appetites

In Greek: μελιτζάνες με φέτα, pronounced meh-leed-ZAH-nes meh FEH-tah

The classic combination of baked eggplant, tomato, and herbs is enhanced by the addition of feta cheese to create a delicious meatless appetizer, side dish, or meatless or main dish.

Cook Time: 45 minutes

Total Time: 45 minutes

Melitzanes me Feta: Baked Eggplant with Feta Cheese

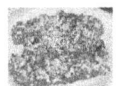

Ingredients:

- 2 pounds of eggplants (long slender type)
- olive oil for frying
- 5 tablespoons of fresh chopped basil
- 5 cloves of garlic, minced
- 1 pound of ripe tomatoes, diced
- 1/2 pound of feta cheese, crumbled
- sea salt
- freshly ground black pepper

Preparation:

Wash the eggplants and remove stems. Cut lengthwise into 1/2 inch slices. Fry lightly (until soft and gently browned) in 1/4 inch of oil.

Preheat the oven to 355°F (180°C).

Layer the eggplant in the bottom of a baking dish. Combine the tomatoes, basil, garlic, and salt and pepper to taste, in a bowl, and spoon the mixture over the eggplant. Top with feta cheese, and bake at 355°F (180°C) for 45 minutes.

Serve hot, warm, or at room temperature.

Summary of exercises.

You must dedicate yourself or rather indulge yourself to these recipes and you will naturally acquire a culinary appreciation of food and be significantly better for it.

In this day and age of our self consuming and busy lifestyle , it is imperative to be practical with our exercises. Remember in our busy lifestyles , home exercises 10 minutes in morning and in afternoon go along way rather than exhausting your body to the point of saturation where the body cannot remain healthy or in balanced weight

This does not mean to make short cuts, but it incorporates, exercise into the context and perspective of lifestyle and not a choir within itself, ineffective by the constant unrealistic pressing on the body to overwork, to only burn out in the end and waste the efforts onto something unnatural.

Jogging once a week can easily be as effective as jogging three times a week.

However because of the omnipresent pollution around us, extra exercise can be a view to precautionary and as a preventative

It incorporates the realities of everyday life. For example walking your dog or on your own is both relaxing to the senses and good for the circulation of your body.

Stretches are mild weight lifting with with lowest threshold of effort and exertion, but with high sustained results when done regularly and therefore is practical to sustain and maintain your fitness.

Recreational exercise eliminates the pressure you exert onto yourself by pushing yourself with the idea of excessive exercises in order to lose weight suddenly and dramatically. But realistically sets it as gradually. For example notice times in your life you lost weight without exercise because of a busy day or that squeezing of the juice was exercise within itself.

It is the idea that you are enjoying yourself by stimulating your brain and senses whilst being social able and forgetting about measuring all that running around, or that impractical self defeating exercise in the gym by constantly looking at the mirror while on the tread mill, waiting and rushing to see results.

This sustains an unhealthy and delimited attitude to your health and diet in general and as a matter of fact separates the idea of dieting with the idea of health , when they should be viewed and practiced inseparably and simultaneously one and the same.

A good metabolism is a balanced one and a balanced one is not categorising lifestyle according to when you are dieting, when you are not, when you are exercising and when you are not.

Almost like a yoyo where one extreme balanced off the other in an almost endless cycle.

Metabolism is also an active lifestyle, it is the willingness to walk, it is the ability to keep busy and not be lazy throughout the day. It is the impetus to think plenty, think of the world around you, reading a paper, it is enjoying a walk in a park and all those things that are natural where once we conform to what is natural—it falls into place. True to yourself and your body.

It encompasses every aspect of your life, the way you think, how you perceive life, how you respond to difficult situations and how you resolve certain issues and problems in your life, how you learn and grow.

Of course this includes reacting in a fashion as not to compensate your inadequate lifestyle with the excessive consumption of food. Feel like a cake, read a paper, still your tummy churning then have some toast with very small amount of butter.

Rather allow this to be the standard by which you measure when at times you have overconsumed or had too much sugar in your food or had battered chicken etc,

your body will signal this disagreement and as a response, we should be predisposed to respond to adjusting our habits and food choices at restaurants and what we buy at the grocery, almost constantly.

But not to the degree where we feel pressure built up as if suppressing our appetite.

Diet fads on two levels are bad

One they ask you to excessively pursue having certain foods over others

Second they do not take into account that diet is an aspect of a healthy lifestyle .

Every now and then we like to binge, but is how we binge and enjoy thoroughly these goodies.

But as we know when we splurge too much on cake and lollies, if anyone unfortunately has ever gone through that, we are still hungry because the body has not been adequately fulfilled and nourished which is essential to understanding the supposed thin girls ability and ease by which they eat well is because by properly fueling their body everyday day, they have the energy and health to go about the day and knowing that latter they will not have a snack and at the same time burning it off while remaining adequately nourished.

It is important to understand that we live in an age of marketing and sales, where claims are branded to lure people to buy a product. They promise an instant cure. The same goes for diet fades. It is in this fashion they sell enough units to make a profit. They are quick to mention exercise and lifestyle, but not in context as the fad diet is based on the false presumption of guaranteed results on its own accord.

And usually we have been conditioned that one product, can heal all our ills, or solve all our problems without effort or self reflection.

This is consumer convenience and the idea that health is not something you buy in a bottle, flags in the face of the diet industry that relies on the 18th century oil snakes oil salesman ideal technique that a bottle with fancy glossy labelling will cure all your ills and make you stronger.

Other examples include the facial cream industry.

Although one may argue that if there were one thing on its own that would make a substantial difference with relatively little effort and a relatively low price, why not.

It is not necessarily bad to buy product that may enhance your looks, but it is a problem when we start to rely on them and overlook the fact that in order to preserve outside beauty we have to have the olive oils, the avocadoes, etc. also it is said that natural aloe vera from the plant is more effective.

In other words there is not one magic cure or bullet, it is the state of things, or the state of your immune system that forms the ability and capacity to fight disease and maintain a healthy outlook and size.

So when we focus on maintaining our health, our resistance to disease and infection grows as by sustaining the immune system through a healthy lifestyle which includes good dieting which essentially is having a balanced regime of foods, knowing when to have fruit after meal to clean your mouth and stomach to help with the digestion as also gelato functions.

Some more unusual reasons why people are overweight and eat plenty is because they may live under a powerlines that induces stress and makes you eat more. Once again be a philosopher or a researcher and know your self and the world around us. There is a nature and principle to things that is always our guide. The natural state of the body is not burgeoning fluctuations of weight but consistent low weight.

Knowing when to ask what oils they use when dining out and ascertaining whether it is worth keeping an empty stomach until you go home or whether deciding to continue ordering the food.

It is about constant monitoring of what you do, but not obsessively, but you know after you have that fast food it makes you sick and heavy, that should be the underlining motivation to opt for the pain of walking a little further to a thai place where there are plenty of vegetables and spices to burn all that fat. Gingers and garlics for example just don't satisfy your taste bud, but gives you the cleaning satisfaction like chillies burning a little in your mouth and cleaning and breaking down all the impurities you have digested before. Acquire a taste for these foods. Be a connoisseur.

It is about having filtered water with coffee, to balance the effects of the coffee which unfortunately has many impurities from the production process that it is exposed to.

Cut softdrinks all together.all this sugar brings about an imbalance in your system by building up your blood sugars insulin, and as a result creates a bloating sensation and reduces the ability of your liver to effectively fit to break down all the fats and toxins that accumulate into your body.

You can also get away with allot by drinking water which cleans allot of impurities out and assists your kidneys.

Pharma detox products are a classic example of this marketing spin. Selling the idea of detox in a product when the whole idea and concept of detox is a lifestyle decision

detoxification

Detoxification is the process of fasting, abstaining, or changing your diet on a regular basis by doing a little at a time with the end result always a big difference without effort because you have effectively conditioned yourself to do this as a habit and therefore is easy to engage as it is second nature.

It is not an idea by putting your self in a cycle of guilt binging and then extreme aversion of food, hence putting you in a cycle of no self control with your lifestyle but once again of consistent accrued little steps that make your platform threshold always that little higher.

It also culminates in the idea that a busy lifestyle, is one that does not see food as the major health issue revolving around your lifestyle needs, it is something in between where you are in a state of preoccupation of life activity and through good times or bad times, forget about eating temporarily until you wait a little day to eat well.

It is making the right decision when to eat and when to drink, like instead of eating a full meal have some bread with that coffee and also save money.

Of course this is not always the way, but if your preparing a great meal that will fill you up latter, why not.

A time to drink and a time to eat, and not to confuse them both, especially when you want a snack, maybe the indulgence of a mocha chino or tea is an activity to defer you from the idea.

Understand the patterns and habits of your behaviours and slowly break these cycles into a lifestyle that is not in accord to preconceived ideas and rules, but according to the natural rhythms of the body.

Adequate intakes of rest and water paramount. It has be shown the benefits of 2 hours rest siesta a day or little cat snaps can substantially improve your energy levels exponentially.

When you are starting out, you will have estranged views of when you are hungry when really you are not. It is ok to go with a hungry stomach but it is good to purposely remain hungry. This is irresponsible.

Little on FAD DIETS

Unbelievable

You have the 1 day diet and the 3 day diet.

As the nature of the commodity is one of being a dispensable disposable consumer able.

In other words, marketing claims to own the solution in a bottle, so to sell that image and sell the concept to you in a bottle.

This is the advent of brand placement in everyday life space. Reducing what is a prerogative and a lifestyle choice of a conscientious health member of society into the false and empty claims of a miracle diet fad that somehow magically you will be skinny and live happily ever after.

Understand the premise of the diet fad. It uses pieces of information that may be true and construes them into a brand product with promises and claims when diet issues form parcel to parcel to the state of your holistic well being and life for example – buying a lemon detox from the pharmacy is comical when one understands the true nature of fasting and detox. This is acquired not through corporate sponsored information but life information.

Being overweight is not a medical condition needed to be treated, it is a result of a deficiency in lifestyle in behaviour and in worldview outlook.

Here is another example of information you should be amicable to.

With the latest news feb 2011 that diet drinks make you more fat.

When people understand how marketing trys to communicate an image and convey a wrongful message through the alluring of promises, images, claims and statements, then one will not only save their money but their energy in focusing on their health rather trying to find a lazy short cut without being in touch with themselves, their attachments and habits etc. because marketers cannot make money on criticising their clients or consumers.

Be aware that we will eventually eat something that disagrees with our body and that it was the food available at the time, when mom made something to conserve money or time but deep frying frozen food, like I had last night.

However it is making the best of a situation, up some salad and complement with fresh water and having herbal tea at night and an apple or fruit in the morning can be that extra little bit at a time, accelerate diet fad that will see results, only with the benefit that as it becomes a lifestyle habit, it will be the constant maintenance of this status quo ideal.

Often we eat something bad and our nature dictates, that we stuffed it up, what is more junk food going to do, or I stuffed it up and lost the new lifestyle diet perspective and I will eat silly and start again at some future juncture.

This negative reinforcement fails to see the role or food and lifestyle as inbuilt defence mechanisms to cater for the times when your body is in disarray from some bad junk food eating incident that you gave into.

Feel the guilt of having that food, but make sure not to give up and see the bigger picture and resolve to try better next time, in a endless cycle of self improvement. This is the essence of anger to motivation. I paid 10 dollars to feel like this after the meal: how long is it going to take to loss this weight??? Knowledge empowers.!!

Remember this built in mechanism of feeling guilty is merely a way our body responds to eating something bad, as a way and inner defence mechanism and signal mechanism that reminds us when we stray. Do not penalise yourself or beat yourself up about these bad incidents, but remember to incrementally improve through firstly a immediate detox strategy after a bad meal so to ease your stomach and digestion and then to refrain from eating this food.

I will be a advocate of saying to avoid certain fast food places all together, but it is not always a reality, I would instead focus on these little detox follow ups and then slowly discover new recipes and foods and even some greek lentil soups eaten with onions shallots and bread.

Remember mistakes will often be repeated and so your ability to make these frequent little fasts, like eating an apple, goes along way beyond what you can imagine and having an apple after a bad meal will help incredibly with mitigating the harmful effects of the bad food experience. Please have this in your arsenal and remember an apple has unreplicatable properties that act medicinally to mitigate toxins and excess fats stored in the body. Do not listen to those that say it is all sugar. This is the middle ages mind set of those who do not know the nature of things

Sometimes it takes quite a few times when you make that decision that you will discipline yourself to have fruit and water after some junk food and then eventually you will cut that junk food and just have the apple.

Sometimes reacting impulsively to a bad eating experience by doing a little exercising or deciding to go to gym can be good, but be wary, that you have to streamlime activity of into a lifestyle of healthy behaviour and actions.

The exercise could be a temporary form of punishment and reminder to walk a little further up the road to thai place and just have plenty of water.

But don't get caught up in this cycle.

Going to a group meeting I thought I'd lavish with myself on lollies, bullets and barbeque flavoured chips

Whenever you eat something that did not agree with you, you should always make a note of it.

Got sick from drinking coffee outside, try to circumvent by alternative days of drinking in nice air conditioned places.

When you cook eggs put plenty of garlic shallots and tomatoes to self clean the food.

When you had too much coffee and feel bloated, watch out for the processed sugar and the milk, inherent complex products your body is working over time to get rid of..

In the morning after scrapping for whatever is in the fridge, I developed a headache.

Someone who has not taken panadol for 5 years, I am someone who always believes we get headaches for a reason and that we need our bodies time to detoxify ourselves from the rubbish we have consumed.

Feeling sticky cold sweats on my skin, it is apparent my immune system is trying to heat allot of it out of my skin through the immune system. I have to not give in to that cheddar cheese. Some call in lachtose intolerance I universalise it by calling it chemical sludge intolerance. Cold sweats and bloated stomach from eating 3-4 slices of this cheese, this is why I insisted my mother buy cottage haloumi or feta cheese, so you can still acquire the benefit. Or even unpasteurised italian cheese or french, if you can afford it. This is cheese with living cultures in them. Most cheeses are processed sludge with insurmountable amounts of salt and are dead black by products like many oils on the market

. Avoiding this food alone goes along way. Learning to replace it can be easy with relatively little pain. Remember that incremental steps make things gradually better. Do not be discouraged if abstinence makes it completely unbearable, be patient with the gradual and the confronting experience will make you more pliable and will change your perspective holistically without artificial induction or inducement

My choice is that by keeping the headache, which given time will go away when my bodies chemistry level returns to its optimum natural level, I would have learnt a lesson to try next time to avoid it or at least to have an apple or more fruit that day as the effects of eating rubbish would not have been so painful In other words, it is the body that signalises us when we need to do more for our health and body and gaining weight works the same way and It is not bad on the onset that we are motivated to eat better just because of our weight. As if this is the one thing that produces fear for you to remain healthy so be it. It is one gauge by which we measure our health and if we see a bit of a belly, well we can be a drastic to the extent of even exercising or completely refraining from the next meal, but latter have a light meal. Don't ever think of bulimic activity , remember this does absolutely nothing , not to mention the danger to your health. Remember it is about solving the underlining root issue of the problem.

However relying solely on having your weight down means being vulnerable to the superficial antics that are involved in keeping weight down and this is the diet fad generation.

Other motivations that should encompass your worrying behaviours of eating wrongly or in excess are avoiding illness, headaches, maintaining immune system, having a clear head to concentrate at work and having a good mood and generally feeling good about yourself.

All these points should encompass to comprise your concerns about your weight, otherwise, u will be susceptible to the easy way out lazy fads promoted in the form of marketable products that are really geared merely to create referral business for the lucrative product placements. Health first and then the rest will take its natural course.

The secret is to feel light and clean . as the taboo phrase goes, beauty starts from the inside.

For the woman you will notice a loss of complexion and youthful appearance when you indulge in artificial flavoured chips. But if you do, it is temporary and through the uses of regular detox strategies immediately after these often inevitable situations, you will maintain health and by engaging is these detox activities, is like a little punishment to yourself not to do it again. But I like to indulge in those chips from time to time. Why not – junk can even relax our stress and nerves. So a balanced lifestyle and diet can accommodate for these foods but in perspective and not to the point where our appetite controls us.

Doing the required work for the required work lost.

Often psychologically we give up when we eat and say to ourselves what is another cake going to make the difference.

To keep in control with your diet, means to let go of trying to control too much, as we are not perfect and we all eat silly things because of the spontaneity of the moment and through each varying situation we confront in our daily lives..

Diet fades are removed and devoid of lifestyle and therefore totally unrealistic.

If the cause of the problem is not addressed ,then masking the symptoms, by surrendering to quick instantaneous solutions via stupendous product claims of weight loss products, will only aggravate your weight problems when you separate weight loss with lifestyle and health.

Excessive skinniness is not a sign of health and this reflects and is noticed by everyone.

Certainly if one cannot discipline herself or himself in eating sultana's and peanuts as snacks, then – have a little bit hard candy, that is mainly comprised on water and sugar.

However if you do not have it in your cupboard, then allow yourself to agonise and agonise and maybe make yourself some greek soup.

Drackahna. Nothing like a soup to replenish your appetite that desired nutrition anyway. So what more better way to satisfy your appetite by replenishing what your body actually desires rather than what you habitually desire and want. That soup great, I am going to sleep.

So now you avoided eating a whole bag of chips which did not satisfy your hunger much but contributed to your belly by restoring the body with proper replenishing food and also enjoying the food at the same time. A double win!!!!!

Do not put stock inside, it is nice as it is. Maybe you just want to put a little.

This should feel your appetite, if not drink something and watch something. But do not let yourself be repressed by trying to control genuine hunger pains, this is just irresponsible.

It is about experience and what I say are simply guides, as everybody have different battles and perceptions however there is one objective truth.

Recognise the internal deficiency in your behaviours rather than outsourcing blame elsewhere, because of the easily available crap in food and the convenient generation mentality of product claims promoting the easy guilt free feeling and irresponsible free indulgence.

One cannot follow a proper course and path to health unless they see the hypocrisy of food processed products and certain medicines that falsely claim instantaneous diet results and making the appropriate action to eating raw foods and preparing them as a cook. You are now going to be a cook, in that way you know you always start with the olive oils, garlics, shallots as primers that activate the gourmet taste to all sorts of meals. You will discern take out places, ask the oils they use, refrain from eating once in a while , whilst being out.

You should know not to add butter even when recipes say too. Of course there are rare exceptions

Getting back to nature and getting back to raw foods is inherently important.

However traditionally it has been through the parameter of culture that we were able to acquire health dishes without effort.

But today in the crude age of commodity based food culture, we have to recognise that treating ourselves to a popular healthy chef dish on t.v. should not be the exemption, but the boring and accessible norm.

It is the nature of things, recognise the difference after eating beans and salad versus paying attention to how we feel after eating meat versus how we feel after eating too much meat and processed garbage..

There is no doubt, when someone pays attention to their body and is in touch with the signals of their immune system that encompasses total holistic health then we are as intuitive geared towards embodying responsible health conscious people, then they will see clearly for what little difference of sacrificing taste for the bean salad, one is astonished at the energy they receive latter as a result and the basic clarity and light feeling they attain as a result from eating better and see clearly it is not just about losing weight but being healthy and having a good healthy lifestyle without free of disease as you are in control of sustaining your immune system with regular eating of the category of foods that are garlics capsicum, chilis and shallots etc.

Practical it is – eating beans with bread and spring onions allows you to get that good fill up feeling, not the soggy chemical greasy fill up feeling you get after eating junk food.

I ask you irritable bowl syndrome or you ate something that your body said no to? Use your common sense and take control of your diet and lifestyle .

Recipe idea.

Prepare spinach and broad beans to boil with little olive oil, then eat this with plenty olive oil, some salt and plenty lemon.

You will be astonishing surprised how enjoyable this meal is with bread and eating alternatively with onions and shallots.

Let food be thy medicine---hippocrates, in the age of patent medicine, appreciating food is not bound and restricted by its taste, but you ought to recognise food inherently for both its taste and health benefits, eg, when you eat certain thai dishes, as long as there is no msg, as you can never be certain what is put in and never be afraid to ask} the enjoyment of food is both its heating cleansing effect which carries its inherent taste and herein lies essentially the culinary appreciation of food.

It not the chemical taste of certain fast food places, but how nature intended the complimentary function of herbs. Etc.

Don't we love the lemon grass in thai and all the vegetables that we do not even notice we are eating.

This is the culinary process of true appreciation and enjoyment of food as a lifestyle benefit both entertaining and both as a medical boaster.

Although legalistic one cannot make that claim, one is burdened with their own discernment and intuition of understanding the commoditized market around them and the products that have came naturally and for free that lie abundantly all around us.

I cannot stress the importance of always eating all foods with salads, whether chips, pasta, steak, everything, fish and chips.

Because in the salad we have the essentials of our health,that can moderate and maintain our health with relatively little effort, but by default to custom, habit and dare I say culture.

In all civilised societies that produced vegetables and fruits in gardens and then entertained guests in the garden, it would have been inconceivable that dining experience would have been merely chips and fish.

With simply egg plant—their can be 10 different types of enjoyable recipes around this powerful and healthy vegetable,

Never say you want something quick and easy like microwave dinners, you must spend time preparing them and preparing you fridge to have the basic ingredients so that you can easily prepare and access them when it is time to cook.

Prepare chips with virgin olive oil as opposed to canola or cotton seed. I cannot stress the importance of oils. Chips with virgin olive oil is truly nutritional and fat free. Learn how different oils are made and distinguish between industrial sludge marketed for consumption and proper eating oils.

Remember restaurants concerned with overheads buy 2nd grade oils.

But this is what god meant for us to be healthy –was through living in harmony with nature in a world now where our natural surrounds have been replaced for the deceitful and confusing concrete jungle, where we have not just lost touch with ourselves, but with how natural food actually tastes, and how to compensate our imbalances through the wonder and miracles of medicinal food.

Also eating these foods in balance and diversity, will more than satisfy our appetites and our satisfaction as , processed food is also eaten to excess because of the deficiency of its nutrients and so –we may still be hungry and dissatisfied intuitively because of this inherent deficiency in junk food.

Where most of it is passed and the body retains very little and all the energy consumed, means you will be hungry again really quickly after eating this garbage.

Remember the gingers, the onions, the spring onions, the mustard, the capsicum, the chilli , the garlics. When adding to beautiful tomatos, paisley and cucumber.

Buy wholegrain pasta if concerned about these carbs. But never shy away from a good warm and fulfilling well cooked meal that will last you the night and from incessant snacking.

What better benefit than adding flavour to your food while receiving the benefit that it maintains your for your immune system

A little more on exercise.

It is so significant as I have inferred and mentioned previously, is the tendency of people to over exercise through gyms when the little rest they do , or the little balance in other activities of their lives, makes the experience artificial and the body so overwhelmed as to the extent that this extreme loss of energy, requires the extreme rejuvenation of energy and the hence the cycle of extremes that simply do not maintain health for the long term and this can manifest inconsistent health regimes that are untenable and therefore we tend to engage in quick diet fixes.

I cannot stress more that by exercising a little in the morning, in small packet intervals and doing 150 skips before the shower and then to work each morning and by enjoying weekly recreation exercise activity that also engages stimulates the mind is more effective than mechanically going to the gym and counting off those calories in front of the mirror. This only puts more untold pressure on yourselves. Of course there are times you have to get out of your comfort zone, however once you frame yourself in habit into a relatively healthy lifestyle, it will be second nature as long as you go through the compensatory actions after when you waver from time to time

The imperative here is the priority of balance in life. Practicality is not inconvenience but the practical means of maintaining yourself at relatively little effort,

which makes sense for a long term strategy.

It is important to emphasise the danger of fade diets as they do not tackle the root cause of the holistic situation of which therein lies and forms the long term solution and cure to obesity in general.

Fad diets inherently by nature, create imbalance.

Operations to change your anatomy, are complete folly and do not address the underlining issues of excessive weight, which is a clear enough signal from your body not to be complacent by trying to find short cuts for the sake of appearances, you have to become it.

If you try to induce the body to chemically think it is full, then you imbalance the body in other ways ,where the body needs to compensate for this. The principles of nature cannot be changed and they are always consistently the same no matter what technology or new product comes to market.

The body will experience fluctuations and symptoms as a result.

Do not fall for the marketing fad and sell up. Research the area of marketing. Understand the philosophy and nature of the body.

Diet exercise,lifestyle etc all play a part and there are no short cuts.

Co ordinated exercises while in a relaxed state

Watching a movie and simultaneously sporadically do leg stretches. Knees curled right up to chest, then release down with legs extending out to the full.

Before shower, knees up to chest whilst lifting up arms up and down.

When you stimulate your intellect with knowledge of how a system works, learning the truth behind the intricate public façade of its propaganda etc is a great way to motivate yourself and find an impetus to our dieting concerns.

We should all feel propelled for something and why not that something be for truth.

Spending too much time with magazines only damages your health and how you view yourself. For me most girls dressing up in those clothes in magazines are too skinny and unhealthy.

Guys don't like those ultra skinny girls on the cat walk anyway, I have asked around.

Of course we like skinny but curvaceous and voluptuous .

Simple stretches right before a shower do plenty as it does not consume your energy for the day to other activities.

The best optimum amount of energy is slightly getting off your comfort zone, and adds a little energy buzz to your particular days activities.

At a café, stretch your arms and hold and feel it in your stomach.

We have to get out of the mind set that exercises are something we do that is separate from life and our daily activities where we recluse to a gym and look at ourselves in the mirror.

It has to be recognised that stretches are form of exercise and weight lifting and a under estimated one. As it builds circulation develops muscles without very little exertion.

It is more productive per energy unit you put in for results than if you were to apply full exertion.

Of course it is important to do full exercise activities but this is better through a social sporting network where you are enjoying yourself while exercising without putting pressure on yourself , if you are losing weight or not.

When walking your dog, do a little bit of running on the spot, 3 times for 30 seconds each time. And once a week, take that walkj through the park to get to that destination with walk and jog and then repeat til you reach destination. The result is a feeling of being more alive, more alert, concentration up, looks up, life up and everything up. This is the inherent reward for exercise.

This preoccupation is not healthy and patience is in order by viewing and seeing it from the perspective of doing a little at a time.

Especially do not be afraid of walking whether your dog or walking to the stores.

This is probably the best form of exercise.

I hope this ebook has inspired you to evaluate your dieting strategies from a point of view of lifestyle and health and not from the point of view of easy way fad schemes and strategies.

So all the best , be vigilant and keep the faith.

Quick pointers

Always arrange snacking with small proportions coupled with fresh water or ginger , camomile tea or peppermint tea.

Pumpkin seeds at night can be a good alleviate of midnight cravings, however do not be afraid to eat late at night because your hungry, it may mean you are truly hungry and your body is desiring replenishment, re nourishment and refuel.

Other reminders are the use of transfatty oils that are entrenched and prevalent with fast food culture. When you think about it, it is this factor alone that makes fast food unhealthy, otherwise what is a bun and a piece of meat and some salad. Once again reaffirming the misconceptions of the product themselves, although they inherently not healthy, it is the chemicals that comprise the food that is naturally hard for the body to break down and wreck havoc for our body , not just our weight but our health. Add on weight is merely a symptom of a state of unhealthiness.

No short cuts allowed in dieting. A lifestyle of food cuisine, partaking and getting involved in the art and philosophy of food culture is paramount. Like that zucchini, or avocado, or cucumber, inherently great beauty foods, you should ask yourself what can be added to these foods to make them appealing because already from the vantage point of improved complexion they give u, they are worth the diet consideration and inclusion. Perhaps you can make up your own recipe.

Remember the main task of cooking is the gathering of the foods. This is exercise within itself and of course anticipation.

Constant self checking and analysing which foods we are taking and which ones are we being deprived of.

The knowledge about how most oils are made and how numerous oils, branded and marketed as natural are infact unnatural and unhealthy and use solvents and dangerous chemicals in the processing.

That is why a little research on products and checks are paramount as they provide a impetus for companies to be on guard with the products they provide the public and therefore are more likely to preserve the quality of their food, because automatically, public knowledge means it is now indispensable to their marketing campaigns.

Oil labelled as pomace oil, is not real oil but is synthesised with chemicals like many other industrial based commercial oils you buy in the supermarket.

Wow . to eliminate this one thing in your diet, goes along way to living a weight light and healthy lifestyle. Complexion mood and all. But information that requires us to be as little philosophers and curious about labelling behind products and the wider knowledge of knowing that we are dealing with an age of processed food where food has been stripped off its nutrition for the sake of the productivity and commodity driven food agriculture , that is seen by business as a commodity and not as a food that is sacred and valuable to the point it needs to be preserved over profits.

If your softdrinking, be sure you can get addicted and all that sugar can bloat you.

Be quick to exchange this with fresh filtered water from tape and invest in a filter. Such as pure water systems, as our thirst is only truly replenished with water and not always softdrinks which are mostly soda and sugar

Some quick other thoughts that are important to note.

A recent article has shown results of how onions burn fat as what I noted before in the ebook, about these types of foods—the garlics, capsicum, the onions etc. especially the use of ginger when your sick is highly useful.

With the recent information in Australia how many producers use human waste for their fertiliser, it is important to go to local markets and make effort in finding quality food.

Although you can never control the pesticides in the food it is important, though, they remain nutritional.

Another tip--- reduced portions of junk food. Or have rice crackers 98% fat free, I find tomato and basil are tasty and have very little bloat factor.

Which claim fat free and no msg etc. beautiful rice crackers.

When we do eat junk it does not nourish our hunger and so we want to eat more, for example when we eat franchised food, allot of it, will make you hungry again latter, because it is no nutritional.

Some other tips

Lift raises of legs during office sit downs and also little on the spot jogs.

Do the trick to give you more energy and do incomparable amount of good with the little energy you put in.

Over exercising is a common fallacy. The right lifestyle for you will mean those little exercises between during and before work for brief 3-5 minute periods are better than long guilt driven exercise bouts where we completely try to get rid of the pounds we gained from a lifestyle that did not accommodate these little habitual and relatively effortless set of exercises and led only in having to gain weight latter and digress to a pattern of weight fluctuations and unmoderated activities of a guide less lifestyle plan .

Because exercise was not part of your normal holistic routine that centred around the motivation and rejuvination of proportional incrementally building energy levels, feelings of better wellbeing, better complexion, disease prevention and general concerns about health in an age of pollution, you centred exercise as a last cry of help, like prayer, when we ought to be praying regularly too and so as a result, we are depleted and burnt out.

. This is a fallacy as it is shown that living a busy lifestyle with exercise in moderation is better than excessive exercise with no breaks.

Also keep in mind—why after eating junk, cakes, biscuits and lollies—why is it we are still hungry—it is because our body has no been properly nourished.

Additional critique and reminder

Processed foods and raw foods we have explored

Acquiring a taste of natural foods and its importance in maintaining health.

Motivated to eat well and restoring appetite for good nutritional food that truly fulfils and satisfies we have covered and I stress its paramount importance as being thin is not a good enough reason , but this is intrinsically linked to being healthy and prudent in your joint lifestyle and eating habits.

Being one of the reasons for excess food, why when we are full we are depleted nutritionally as we still want to eat.

This phenomena can be seen with many fast foods. I have spoken about this and this gets into food philosophy and the reason for people having good metabolisms is because they eat nutritionally filled food properly where they have no need to eat again latter in the night and know how to control themselves.

If in the morning you are bloated , let it be a lesson and have a little detox. Have some fruit and water and even better peppermint tea. Exercises don't do any harm but they make you feel better anyway by having more energy and having more endurance and agility. Also feeling better how you look. Of course it is ok for weight increase to act within a motivation within itself to change.

As it is the one noticeable marker showing a deficiency in a lifestyle or eating habit. But one should never be carried away but rather put into perspective and take the appropriate course of action.

Firstly by bad food avoidance as we all know there is a consequence of a bloat we instinctual feel after that slice of cake for example.

This acts to urge us as a reminder before we are tempted again, that avoidance will make us feel better an cleaner and more in control. It is important to know that eating in moderation junk is ok as they do comprise some of the delights in nature's arsenal.

For example, home-made cakes can still be very healthy or certain delicacy, but remember the fat is usually because of some chemical or by natur e of a complex compound food.

There are numerous research articles centred around the role of trans fat, processed foods, industrial sludge fake oils and general food additives and chemicals that contribute to fat.

But do not feel hopeless about it, becaue remember the apples, the tomatoes are so rich with anti oxidants that thy will neutral the bad ingredients we may partake in our dishes and servings. We are going back to the idea of little compensations again that lead to a consensus of good food mitigation practices that sustain your immune system, keep you healthy and build your resistance and tolerance to possible future episodes of food poisoning.

Chedder cheese is a great example of a food, where the oils and the chemicals used in the food is what gives you the instant bloat and unhealthy feeling. However in moderation it is still ok. Please remember the cheese and oils. Research them because it is not hard to eliminate these foods or fake foods.

The idea of an occasional fast food burger is fine and better without chips, because the oils they use are completely unnatural whether soy cotton oil and many other branded vegetable oils with transfatty acids

It is not the content of the food that usually makes you fat, but the chemicals.

Creating turmoil in your gut culture, complex compounds find it difficult to digest, leading to excess weight.

Eating fruit after food is paramount, not only will this avoid you going to the dentist with potential evasive and unnecessary dangerous treatment, but you will keep your health.

The state of your mouth and teeth are always a really good gauge of your nutrition.

If after a meal you have bad breathe, there is nothing like having an apple to regain that clean and satisfied feeling knowing your doing good for your digestion, health and complexion and most importantly your mouth culture environment and revitalising your essential stomach gut culture to its normal metabolic rate and capacity. This is our reassurance when we eat on occasion too much, that If we keep our gut healthy then it has a greater propensity to deal with waste and toxins that you consume. This is the confiding and beautiful metabolism , even when you start out and resort to old eating routines that are damaging to your health, you will do a great deal to your health by just ingesting filtered water and fruit afterwards. That is the power of fruit.

This unfortunate oversight aspect of food culture is a product of a generation in the western world that lost touch with themselves their own nature and who adopted to fatalistic perverted ideas of fast food and instant gratification, losing your taste for the finer more natural foods because of our indifferent indulgence in un nutritional fast food.

We identify a headache or onset on a sore stomach as something spontaneous or random that has nothing to do with our behaviour. This is the major obstacle to overcome to be able to surrender and immerse yourself into this lifestyle. This is the way you see life. If you do not take responsibility for your actions and practice diligence and frugality and moderation then far from the philosopher we are constantly in anxiety to satisfy and quench our passions of which we have no control in our lives and that act as a parasite, where we ask the basic question, how can we look forward to junk when we have it all the time. Sometimes deprivation is healthy for the mind and body and this innately reacts a cleaning process within our bodies, that is exhausted with all the meat and cheese we consume everyday.

Monitoring our energy levels, do we feel chronically tired, this means we need to on occasion sacrifice that morning coffee with little milk and have a fresh orange juice, not processed orange juice. But if you economising then buy the 100% juice at the shops, it is much better than the softdrinks. But softdrinks are a great refresher especially the chinoto italian softdrinks as they come in small servings as well, so we do not rely on them to quench our thirst, this should be reserved for water.

Always take fruit with you. Have a piece of fruit in the morning and no toast. But have your big egg and bacon breakfast on weekend. Eggs are so nutritional , do not even think that its fat content, it is inconsequential if you are eating a general balancing lifestyle, as the marginal fat content of the egg is balanced and averaged off by your lifestyle.as a matter of fact the egg and bacon on the weekend is a energy boaster for your lifestlye as you need now to carry on this metabolism rate as this requires energy. Now the high metabolic girl myth is explained.

Your lifestyle ought to revolve around prepared social engagements, sport engagements, time for reading or a hobby. cake free coffee time. Times when we should be drinking rather than eating as we mentioned before. Pushing your comfort zone once a day but never more. Proportional is better than cold turkey.

Take a walk after work, try to fill your day with some friends and also time for self reflection and bedroom exercises as we spoke about

Can you eat a carrot and a tomato on its own?

Can you find a tomato, olive, cucumber, haloumi, garlic and carrot celery platter as being a pleasurable snack. You will be surprised when you refind your natural appetite that naturally and instictually likes these foods, then you will easily resort to these foods as avenues of pleasure, as you at this point will know that a cake would have still made you hungry latter and we spoke about that early on.

Acquiring the taste, especially of a tomato really goes along way, as it is not about different people having different tastes, the taste of an apple and tomato are universal and so when people dislike tomatoes, it may well be a personal justified conviction, however from a universal perspective they have failed to acquire a taste for a vegetable or a fruit as some call it , that plays an integral role in salads that in turn plays an integral part to your compliment servings with chickens and steaks as it self cleans and compliments your meals on a deep and profound level. If one were close to nature and one loves nature how can they dislike the fruits that grow from nature-- this is the philosophical outlook.

. Usually those who dislike tomatoes don't like salads.

They loss how onions and shallots and ginger mixed in with a tuna salad for example, compliment to taste of the salad as a whole, creating that exquisite gourmet taste and also having a the onions and shallots acting as the cleaners with the salad as well of course the balsamic vinegar, olive oil and lemon. There is nothing like it. Having bread to fill you up is a great idea. But remember the best bread are the ones non gluten natural breads

So enjoy. Observe, remain vigilant with what you eat, this is not a superficial weight things, most woman who are in control know this –it is also about how good whole foods stabilise your moods, give you positive vibes , help you to remain focused and healthy during the day and keeps your complexion great like no other expensive over marketed cream will. There is no short cuts and this is the new food philosophy slash lifestyle. Don't be lazy. Work a little everyday

.

lastly we have a little information on health tonics that will boast your energy and will further incline you away from snacking.

Remember it is about listening to the signals and the cues of the body that act intelligently and seek balance.

When we cough the body tries to get rid of the toxin stuck in our bodies. We should aid it not suppress it. When we have a sore stomach, what did you eat and what was in the food that you usually take for granted. Do you take headache tablets often. Why? Don't you know that this is a sign of deficiency in your body, but you ask what does this have to do with weight loss and my health. I will say it is not just related, it is everything. An apple after each meal will see you cutting your intake of headache tablets by half. This is the lifestyle we acquire as philosophers trying to find balance in proportion and happiness with contentment and moderation not through excess as this is not real happiness.

Is their a drug perscribed making you more sick or fluctuate and more fat, look for a second opinion and look for alternatives. Remember nature has provided for all and modern science has got too much of the credit as being the saviour for man.

It was not penicillin that saved man from the germ infested world of infection and death, but the improved sanitation conditions introduced in the beginning of the 19th century.

One thing we take when we observe our love for softdrink is the constant awareness is evokes that it is not really replenishing us but is simply gutting our gut. These are the integral signs by which we act and never be lazy and so if you must have a soft drink take it but then follow your thirst with water and so you are incrementally adjusting and improving within balance and with relative ease and effort.

Lastly the last note is on cosmetics and appearances.

Why do we constantly dry out our sculp with the overuse of shampoos and conditioners ??

this is another area where we are conditioned to believe we need to clean our hair everyday. This is a fallacy. Of course the companies of shampoos want you to buy more without allowing you to observe the damage you are doing to your hair from overuse of shammpoos and conditioners that are heavily laden with toxic chemicals .

In the greco roman medical texts there is the emphasise of using hair tonics to maintain the youthfulness and vibrancy of your hair.

Replenishing our hair with essential oils and and even extra virgin olive oil.

Use essential oils in your life. Cucumber for your eyes, eat some avocado before a dinner date, eating salads before an outing will give you that extra complexion.

Right now I am feeling a bloat from the extra chiptotle sauce put in my veg dellite as subway.

This is the best fastfood as long as you get all the salads, more than what we would probably stock at home. The chilis and pickles and onions are cancelling out the sauce and cheese-- so for me I compensate the lack of nutrition derived from the cheese with the burning and cleaning properties of all those salad ingredients. Processed meats are bad. Avoid as much as you can. All the best and keep a diary and plan your life. God bless and god loves you.

On Tonics. Energy and weight loss

3. Honey and Lemon: Weight Loss Diet Tip
A honey and lemon diet can relieve you of your weight problem. Find out why more and more people are trying out this Honey and Lemon Diet Tip.

4. Milk and Honey: For promotion of good digestion and health
Adding honey to diary products such as sour milk and yoghurts can improve your digestion and bowel movements. Read more about what is so good about Milk and Honey.

Hippocrates treated his patients with Apple Cider and Julius Caesar's army used ACV to stay healthy and fight off disease. The Greeks and Romans kept vinegar vessels for healing and flavoring, and Samurai warriors drank it for strength and power.

Apples contain a host of beneficial vitamins and minerals, such as phosphorous, potassium, magnesium, calcium, iron, and many trace elements as well. Apples are the main ingredient in Cider vinegar making it a powerful detoxifying and purifying agent.

Organic Apple cider vinegar is a completely natural product with amazing health benefits.

In production it is twice fermented. The first stage is from apple juice to apple cider followed by a second fermentation to apple cider vinegar.

The extra acids and enzymes produced during the two fermentation steps make this natural remedy a very nutritional product and an excellent health tonic.

It's the sum of all these ingredients that give ACV it's amazing health benefits.

OXYMEL

04/26/2011: Jc from Savannah, Georgia writes: "I had learnt a while back that the ancient Greeks used to make a drink from vinegar or old wine (vinegar :D), honey and water; it was called Oxymel.

I used to make this drink and with some ice cubes, it's a refreshing and delicious drink. One must experiment to get the taste right and I don't remember the exact recipe I used. Still this may be a good way of getting both ACV and (local) honey in together.

Here is some info on Oxymel: http://heml.mta.ca/wiki/index.php/Oxymel

Another way I found to take it was to add ACV to "organic" apple juice; you don't taste the ACV this way; it tastes only like apple juice."

Sparkling Lemon/Ginger Detox Tonic Recipe:

(As always- adjust levels to suit your taste and use organic when possible- detoxing with pesticide residue doesn't make sense, does it?)

- Juice of Half Lemon
- 1 1/2 teaspoon agave nectar or honey
- 1 1/2 teaspoon chopped ginger, mashed
- 6 mint leaves or 2 lemon verbena leaves
- 10 ounces seltzer or filtered clean water (if you prefer a still tonic)

Muddle ginger with lemon (you can keep the peels on if you want the extra flavor). Add fresh mint or lemon verbena to mixture and muddle until leaves are bruised and torn.

Stir in agave or honey until fully incorporated. Top with seltzer (careful here it can get really fizzy!) You can also use still filtered water if you don't like the bubbles.

Thankyou I hope you enjoyed the ebook and you find happiness with your newly acquired lifestyle and weight.

You can shop and find motivation to lose weight so that you look good in that dress your considering to buy. But remember, no model crap, eat well . being too skinny is out and guys don't like it. Be healthy be happy..

And please remember the natural essential oils – be close to nature and your heart. God bless.

Nicholas lazarou